Gastric Sleeve Cookbook

The Complete Bariatric Recipes Guide & Cookbook for you after Weight Loss Surgery – With Over 110 Recipes

Sarah McCabe

Copyright Legal Information

Table of Contents

Introduction

Thank you for purchasing the Gastric Sleeve Cookbook. The recipes it contains are designed around the different dietary stages you will go through as you recover from surgery. They will ease you into each stage and ensure that you are provided with healthy food that is also delicious.

After your surgery there is a significant adjustment period as your body becomes used to a lower intake of calories, and a limited absorption of energy. This means that making the right choices in what you do choose to eat is incredibly important. The recipes in this book provide the most effective ways to get the nutrients you require in order to make this adjustment as simple as possible.

The next few pages will provide you with more details on the way your diet will be affected, what to expect, and how to address any problems that may arise. It's likely that there will be difficult moments, so don't become disheartened. By reading through the information in this book first, you will be in a better position to take care of yourself as you adjust to life with a bariatric sleeve.

After Your Bariatric Surgery

Immediately after surgery, you will be on a clear liquid diet. This moves to full liquids, soft pureed foods, soft foods, then eventually regular, albeit smaller, meals.

While you are on a clear liquid diet, your body is simultaneously very low in a hormone called ghrelin. This is because the part of the stomach that produces most of this hormone has been removed. Ghrelin is responsible for initiating a hunger response in the body, so even though you are on a very limited diet, you shouldn't find yourself too affected by it.

Make sure that you are consuming liquids in small amounts repeatedly throughout the day. This includes lots of water, and things like broth and decaffeinated tea. Sugar and caffeine must be avoided at this time, so make sure that you are choosing the sugar-free varieties of anything else you do wish to drink. Do not drink any carbonated beverages.

People will experience some pain, but this is most likely to be bearable. You will have painkillers to help with this. There are often ongoing psychological changes, too. Rapid weight loss is attributed to a drastic change in the hormone levels in your body. The people around you should be made aware that you might be more susceptible to mood swings and fatigue.

As you recover and eating becomes less difficult and more appealing again, you become exposed to the risk of overeating. Like any surgery, you are less likely to be hungry immediately following the operation, but recovery makes you feel more and more like your old self, and sets you up to begin eating the way your old self did, too. It's not hard to see why this is a problem, but it comes with a new set of issues once you have had bariatric surgery.

Since your stomach is not only around four ounces in volume, it doesn't take much to fill up. Imagine roughly what would fit in the palm of your hand. If you eat more that this, you are likely to need to vomit in response, and this is just one problem. Acid reflux is common, where extra food gets pushed up the throat in an absence of space. Combined with stomach acids, this is deeply unpleasant and has been attributed to choking in some cases. Another effect, known as 'dumping' is where minimally processed foods get put directly into the small intestine. This can cause cramping and diarrhea, sweating and even fainting. The most significant side effect, though, is stomach stretching. Even after surgery, your stomach can stretch again if you eat too much, putting you at risk of eating more calories than you need, and regaining your weight as a result.

The best way to avoid overeating is to remain constantly mindful of the eating process. Start by ordering smaller portions, and as you eat, constantly monitor your fullness. Chew slowly, take small bites, avoid liquids while eating and always ask yourself whether or not you are truly still hungry. Leaving food on the plate is not a sin, and eating more than you really need will do you no favors.

Food Dos and Don'ts

Do

The main dietary rule to follow post surgery is **high protein, low carbohydrate**. Favouring these foods that are nutrient-dense is how you are going to be able to make the most of the little food you are able to consume, giving your body as much nutrition as possible.

Foods that are best for achieving this goal are **lean proteins like chicken and fish, vegetables, and legumes**. **Eggs and soft cheeses** are also effective ways of delivering these things. They should all be prepared according to the stage of recovery you are in -- be this pureed or in their full form.

Many people also supplement their diet with extra vitamins to make sure the body is getting the nutrition their bodies need, make sure to ask your doctor about this.

Don't

Your diet will become relatively normal once you have fully recovered, but in the beginning there are a few things that should be **avoided completely: sugar, caffeine and spicy foods.** These can be reintroduced in small amounts later, but it is important to speak with your doctor about it.

Long-term, continue to avoid foods that are not dense with nutrients. This means processed foods, concentrated sugars (sweets, for example), and too many carbohydrates. Cook your foods in the healthiest way possible. It will be much harder to process fats, so fried foods are no advised.

Alcohol will be processed differently as well, and while you can start enjoying it again, it should be in smaller volumes as the surgery will often quicken alcohol's effects.

What are Your Health Goals

While bariatric surgery is designed for weight loss, it's important to take a healthy approach to how quickly this happens. Many people find that they begin losing weight almost immediately, with the general trend being that people lose 60% of their excess weight.

It is important to recognize that this is not your total weight, but the weight on top of what would be a healthy weight for you. So, if your ideal weight is 120 pounds, and you weigh 300 pounds, you are expected to lose 60% of 180 pounds, that is, your excess weight.

The food you eat is central to seeing these results, and keeping them. The problem many people encounter is that their lives with the sleeve start to feel incredibly normal, and they have lost a lot of weight, so feel less inclined to restrict their diet. Whether this be by over eating, or consuming calorie-dense foods with now nutritional value, they start to put on weight again.

Your health goal should not be motivated by a goal weight. Everyone is different, and no one's weight loss can be measured by another's. Instead, try to make your goal something you can measure in protein and calories. As a rough guide, **aim for 65-75 grams of protein a day**, and keep your daily caloric intake to **below 1000**. These numbers are general, and your doctor may have a plan more specific to you. If you adhere to them as much as possible, you will continue to see results.

By eating three healthy meals a day, drinking at least 64 oz. of water, and staying vigilant, this should be perfectly achievable. You can use the recipes in this book to make your own meal plans so that you have a better idea of what you should be eating when, which will help you avoid eating things outside of your plan, and therefore intake goals.

Four Phases of the Gastric Sleeve Diet

Breaking your eating habits into these phases allows you to slowly reintroduce solid food into your diet. The timeframes given are an indication only -- make sure to follow your doctor's post-operative instructions to ensure you are tailoring your recovery to you. These lists are an indication only, there may be other things you are able to eat, but again it is best to check with your doctor.

Clear Liquids

Week 1-2 after surgery

This part of the diet is simple in that you are heavily restricted both in what you can eat, and how much you actually feel like eating. Many do not have an appetite but most people will experience above average thirst. The only things you can have at this stage are:

- Broth
- Decaffeinated tea
- Sugar-free popsicles

Your caloric intake should be quite low at this stage, around 200-400 calories per day. Make sure you are consuming plenty of water, in small sips throughout the day. Aim for 64 oz. per day.

Full Liquids

1-2 weeks after clear liquids

This stage is slightly more difficult, as you've now recovered and will start to get your appetite back. You may experience hunger pains as you will not be able to derive the satisfaction you normally get from eating solid foods. It's incredibly important to stay vigilant, however, as your body is in no way ready to process solids. The things you can have at this stage are:

- Protein powder shake (with a sugar-free, non carbonated liquid)

13

- Sugar-free yogurts, puddings, sorbets
- Thin soups (very soft noodles can be added)
- Thinned sugar-free oatmeal
- Sugar-free juice
- Fat-free milk

Soft Pureed Foods

1-4 weeks after full liquids

At this stage you can start focussing on getting your protein intake up. You should be aiming for around 60 grams per day. If you struggle to make this every day, don't become disheartened -- the most important to do is keep trying. Introduce things in small quantities initially, and take note of any foods your body doesn't respond well to. At this stage you can start introducing:

- Hummus
- Mashed potatoes
- Soft cereals, vegetables, and cheeses
- Scrambled eggs
- Tofu
- Tinned fish
- Mashed fruit

Soft Foods and More

Ongoing

This is where you can start enjoying the things you love to eat again. The important things to consider is if you are getting enough protein and nutrients, as well as keeping your sugar intake low. Continuing to drink protein shakes is a good way of getting more into your diet if you are finding it hard to meet your target.

There are still a few things to take into consideration:

- Vegetables should still be cooked until they are slightly soft. Nuts should be avoided

- Fried foods should be avoided
- Sugary, caffeinated, and carbonated drinks should be avoided
- Meats need to be chewed thoroughly
- Whole-fat dairy products should be avoided

Gastric Sleeve FAQs

How can I ensure I am getting the nutrients I need?

In terms of your diet, you should be aiming to eat as many whole foods as possible, changing the types of meats and vegetables you are eating in order to get the maximum amount of vitamins and nutrients.

You can also use supplements to ensure that you are getting everything you need, but you should check this with your doctor.

How many meals can I eat per day?

It is recommended that you eat three small meals a day. You should stop consuming liquids 30 minutes prior to eating to allow a maximum amount of space in your stomach for the nutrients you will be giving it.

At times, such as at restaurants, you may have more food than you need. Make sure that you don't try and finish everything, as this could have unpleasant physical results. Try asking for a half serve, or seeing if anyone would be willing to share a meal with you instead.

Can I eat snacks?

While it's recommended that you adhere to the three-meal-a-day rule, you may experience hunger in between meals. As long as you are eating the right things to address the hunger, you can allow yourself to snack a small amount between meals.

Choosing a combination of high-fiber and high-protein snacks is the best way to snack efficiently. This means things like fruits and vegetables, paired with nut butters, cheeses, and yogurts.

What if I don't feel full?

This is a challenge you will need to overcome as you recover from surgery. As you just read, snack are okay, but if you are relying too heavily on them, you may need to take a more psychological approach when you are eating, to avoid problems when you aren't:

- Concentrate on every mouthful. Chew your food at least 25 times before swallowing, and take small breaks between mouthfuls.
- Constantly assess the way your body feels. Is it hunger, or simply a desire to eat?
- Decide that you are going to stop, and stick to it. Use your brain to master your body. This cannot be learned overnight, rather it's the result of many weeks or months of training.

Another thing to keep in mind is your water intake. If you keep this up throughout the day, your stomach will be fuller more often. While it's not full of food, it will send a message to the brain that it isn't empty, which may help alleviate some feelings of hunger.

Gastric Sleeve Fluids Recipes

Beef and Seaweed Stock

Serving: 8

Total time taken: 45 minutes

Ingredients

- 8 oz lean ground beef
- 1 oz dried seaweed
- 5 cups water
- 2 cloves garlic
- Salt
- Cooking spray

Directions

1. Soak seaweed for 10 minutes. Chop and set aside.

2. Coat a large pot with cooking spray. Over medium heat, saute the garlic. Add in the ground beef and brown.

3. Once meat is browned, add water and bring to a boil. Cover, reduce heat, and simmer for 15 minutes. Skim fat layer that will form on the surface.

4. Add seaweed to the pot. Simmer for 10 more minutes.

5. Strain to remove all solids, keeping only the broth.

6. Refrigerate stock overnight. Remove layer of fat formed before use.

Pork Rib and Bean Stock

Serving: 4

Total time taken: 60 minutes

Ingredients

- 12 oz lean pork spareribs
- 6 oz bean sprouts
- 3 cups water
- 2 cloves garlic (minced)
- 2 slices fresh ginger
- 1 green onion (chopped)
- Salt
- Cooking spray

Directions

1. In a large pot, bring 3 cups of water to a boil. Blanch the pork for 5 minutes. Discard the water.

2. Add 3 cups of fresh water, pork, onion, ginger, and garlic to the pot and bring to a boil. Reduce to low heat.

3. Cover and simmer for 30 minutes. Skim fat layer that will form on the surface.

4. Add bean sprouts to the pot and simmer for 10 minutes.

5. Strain to remove all solids, keeping only the broth.

6. Refrigerate stock overnight. Remove layer of fat formed before use.

Vegetable Fish Stock

Serving: 12

Total time taken: 60 minutes

Ingredients

- 1 lb fish bones (from bass, flounder, or halibut)
- 7 cups water
- 1 onion (chopped)
- 3 slices ginger root
- 4 stalks celery (chopped)
- 2 tablespoons black peppercorns
- 2 tablespoons fresh parsley (chopped)
- 2 tablespoons fresh thyme (chopped)
- 1 bay leaf
- Salt

Directions

1. In a large pot, add water and bring to a boil. Add fish bones and ginger, boiling for 10 minutes.

2. Add celery and onion. Cook for 5 minutes. Add thyme, parsley, bay leaf, and peppercorns, and salt.

3. Reduce to low heat, and cover. Simmer for 40 minutes.

4. Strain to remove all solids, keeping only the broth.

5. Refrigerate stock overnight. Remove layer of fat formed before use.

Bok Choy Stock

Serving: 4

Total time taken: 60 minutes

Ingredients

- 12 oz bone-in chicken
- 3 cups water
- 1 green onion (chopped)
- ½ pound bok choy
- Salt

Directions

1. In a large pot, bring water and chicken to a boil.

2. Reduce to low heat, cover, and simmer for 40 minutes. Skim off fat layer that will form on the surface.

3. Add bok choy and green onion. Simmer for another 10 minutes.

4. Strain to remove all solids, keeping only the broth.

5. Refrigerate stock overnight. Remove layer of fat formed before use.

Vegetable Beef Stock

Serving: 12

Total time taken: 60 minutes

Ingredients

- 1 pound lean beef shank (diced)
- 7 cups water
- 2 slices fresh ginger
- 2 carrots (chopped)
- ½ radish (chopped)
- Salt

Directions

1. In a large pot, saute the onion until fragrant. Add beef and water, bringing to a boil.

2. Reduce to low heat, cover, and simmer for 40 minutes. Skim off fat layer that will form on the surface.

3. Add carrots, radish, and salt. Simmer for another 10 minutes.

4. Strain to remove all solids, keeping only the broth.

5. Refrigerate stock overnight. Remove layer of fat formed before use.

Fishy Tomato Broth

Serving: 12

Total time taken: 60 minutes

Ingredients

- 1 lb fish bones (from bass, flounder, or halibut)
- 7 cups water
- 1 block silken tofu (cubed)
- 2 cups tomatoes (finely chopped)
- 4 slices ginger root
- Salt

Directions

1. In a large pot, add water and bring to a boil. Add fish bones and ginger, boiling for 10 minutes.

2. Add tomatoes and tofu. Reduce to low heat and cover. Simmer for 40 minutes.

3. Strain to remove all solids, keeping only the broth.

4. Refrigerate stock overnight. Remove layer of fat formed before use.

Pork and Fuzzy Gourd Broth

Serving: 12

Total time taken: 90 minutes

Ingredients

- 1 pound pork bones
- 8 cups water
- ½ cup black eyed peas
- 3 medium fuzzy gourd (cut in 1" pieces)
- ½ cups peanuts
- Salt

Directions

1. Soak the peanuts and peas in water for 15 minutes.

2. In a large pot, bring water to a boil. Blanch the pork bones for 5 minutes. Discard the water.

3. Add 8 cups of fresh water, pork bones, peanuts, and peas to the pot. Bring to a boil and reduce heat.

4. Cover and simmer for 30 minutes. Skim fat layer that will form on the surface.

5. Add gourd sprouts to the pot and simmer for 30 minutes.

6. Strain to remove all solids, keeping only the broth.

7. Refrigerate stock overnight. Remove layer of fat formed before use.

Rosemary Grapefruit Infused Water

Serving: 10

Total time taken: 8 hours

Ingredients

- ½ grapefruit (peeled and sliced)
- 1 sprig fresh rosemary
- 4 cups water
- Liquid stevia, to taste

Directions

1. In a sealable jar, add water, rosemary, and grapefruit.

2. Cover and refrigerate for at least 8 hours.

3. Remove all solids from the jar.

4. Add liquid stevia to desired taste before serving. Serve cold.

Citrus Infused Green Tea

Serving: 8

Total time taken: 8 hours

Ingredients

- 2 green tea bags
- 1 lemon (sliced)
- ½ grapefruit (peeled and sliced)
- 4 cups water
- Liquid stevia, to taste

Directions

1. I In a sealable jar, add water, tea bags, lemon, and grapefruit.

2. Cover and refrigerate for 4 hours. Remove tea bags and refrigerate for 4 more hours.

3. Remove all solids from the jar.

4. Add liquid stevia to desired taste before serving. Serve cold.

Spicy Infused Cucumber Water

Serving: 8

Total time taken: 8 hours

Ingredients

- ½ jalepeno (deseeded)
- 1 cucumber (sliced)
- 1 sprig mint leaves
- 4 cups water

Directions

1. I In a sealable jar, add water, cucumber, mint, and jalepeno.

2. Cover and refrigerate for 8 hours.

3. Remove all solids from the jar.

4. Serve cold.

Gastric Sleeve Puree Recipes

Spicy Tofu Puree

Serving: 4

Total time taken: 20 minutes

Ingredients

- 12oz block steamed silken tofu
- ½ teaspoon garlic powder
- ½ teaspoon chili powder
- ¼ teaspoon tumeric
- ¼ teaspoon garlic powder
- ½ teaspoon salt
- 1 tablespoon olive oil

Directions

1. In medium sized pot, bring a few inches of water to a boil. Add tofu to a steaming basket.

2. Cover and steam until cooked, about 15 minutes.

3. In a blender, add steamed tofu and spices.

4. Blend until smooth, adding water or olive oil to reach desired consistency.

5. Serve warm as a side dip.

Spicy Cauliflower Puree

Serving: 2

Total time taken: 20 minutes

Ingredients

- 2 cups broccoli (chopped)
- 2 cups cauliflower (chopped)
- 1 tablespoon olive oil
- ½ cup skim milk
- 1 teaspoon dry mint (ground)
- 1 tablespoon fresh parsley (chopped)
- ½ teaspoon italian seasoning
- ¼ teaspoon ground cumin
- ½ teaspoon salt

Directions

1. In a deep pot, cover cauliflower with water and a pinch of salt. Cook for 15 minutes. Drain.

2. Add cooked cauliflower, broccoli, milk, salt, italian seasoning, mint, parsley, and cumin to the food processor.

3. Blend slowly, while gradually adding olive oil, until thoroughly pureed.

4. Serve with fresh celery and carrots, as desired.

Cauliflower and Beef Puree

Serving: 4

Total time taken: 30 minutes

Ingredients

- 8 oz lean ground beef
- ¾ cup chicken broth
- ½ cup cauliflower (chopped)
- 1 tablespoon fresh parsley (chopped)
- 1 tablespoon fresh thyme (chopped)
- 1 clove garlic (minced)
- Salt
- Cooking spray

Directions

1. In a medium pot of boiling water, blanch cauliflower until soft, about 10-15 minutes. Set aside.

2. Coat a skillet with cooking spray. Over medium heat, add the ground beef and brown.

3. Once meat is browned, add half of the chicken broth and herbs. Cover and simmer for 20 minutes.

4. In a blender, add cauliflower and cooked beef with the broth.

5. Blend until smooth, adding the remaining chicken broth to reach desired consistency.

6. Strain the puree to remove large pieces. Serve warm.

Italian Style Chicken Puree Soup

Serving: 4

Total time taken: 20 minutes

Ingredients

- 8 oz boiled chicken breast (shredded)
- ¼ cup parmesan cheese (grated)
- 1 cup chicken broth
- ½ teaspoon garlic powder
- 1 tablespoon oregano
- 1 clove garlic
- 1 tablespoon fresh parsley (chopped)
- Salt

Directions

1. In a medium sized pot, cover chicken with water and bring to a boil. Cook until done, about 15 minutes.

2. In a separate saucepan, heat the chicken broth.

3. In a blender, add cooked chicken, half of the chicken broth, and all other ingredients.

4. Blend until smooth, adding the remaining broth until desired consistency is reached.

5. Strain the puree to remove large pieces. Serve warm.

Hearty Beef and Potato Puree

Serving: 6

Total time taken: 30 minutes

Ingredients

- 8 oz lean ground beef
- ¼ cup carrot (chopped)
- ¼ cup potatoes (chopped)
- ¼ cup canned pumpkin puree
- 2 tablespoons cheddar cheese (shredded)
- 1 cup chicken broth
- 1 teaspoon tomato paste
- 1 clove garlic
- 1 tablespoon parsley (chopped)
- Salt
- Cooking spray

Directions

1. Coat a saucepan with cooking spray. Over medium heat, saute carrots and potatoes for about 4 minutes.

2. Add the ground beef to the saucepan and brown. Once meat is browned, add in the parsley, garlic, pumpkin puree, tomato paste, salt, and half of the chicken broth.

3. Cover and simmer for 20 minutes. Towards the end, stir in the cheese.

4. In a blender, add all ingredients. Blend until smooth, adding remaining chicken broth to reach desired consistency.

5. Strain the puree to remove large pieces. Serve warm.

Chicken and Pumpkin Puree

Serving: 4

Total time taken: 20 minutes

Ingredients

- 8 oz boiled chicken breast (shredded)
- ¼ cup cheddar cheese (shredded)
- 1 cup skim milk
- ½ cup canned pumpkin puree
- ½ teaspoon Dijon mustard
- 1 tablespoon fresh chives (chopped)
- Salt

Directions

1. In a medium sized pot, cover chicken with water and bring to a boil. Cook until done, about 15 minutes.

2. In a separate saucepan, heat the chicken broth.

3. In a blender, add cooked chicken, pumpkin puree, skim milk, cheese, mustard, chives, salt, and half of the chicken broth.

4. Blend until smooth, adding the remaining broth until desired consistency is reached.

5. Strain the puree to remove large pieces. Serve warm.

Italian Tomato Puree

Serving: 6

Total time taken: 30 minutes

Ingredients

- 12 oz lean ground beef
- ½ cup chicken broth
- 1 cup tomatoes (crushed)
- 2 tablespoon parmesan cheese
- 1 clove garlic
- 1 bay leaf
- 1 teaspoon oregano
- 1 tablespoon fresh thyme (chopped)
- ¼ cup carrot (chopped)
- ¼ cup onion (chopped)
- Salt
- Cooking spray

Directions

1. Coat a saucepan with cooking spray. Over medium heat, saute the carrots and onion until fragrant.
2. Add the ground beef to the saucepan and brown. Once meat is browned, add in the tomatoes, oregano, thyme, garlic, bay leaf, salt, and half of the chicken broth.
3. Cover and simmer for 20 minutes. Towards the end, add in the parmesan.
4. In a blender, add all ingredients. Blend until smooth, adding remaining chicken broth to reach desired consistency.
5. Strain the puree to remove large pieces. Serve warm.

Thai Style Chicken Blended Puree

Serving: 4

Total time taken: 20 minutes

Ingredients

- 8 oz boiled chicken breast (shredded)
- 1 cup chicken broth
- 1 clove garlic
- 1 tablespoon soy sauce
- 1 tablespoon green onion (chopped)
- 2 tablespoons fresh ginger (grated)
- ¼ cup powdered peanut butter
- ½ teaspoon vinegar

Directions

1. In a medium sized pot, cover chicken with water and bring to a boil. Cook until done, about 15 minutes.

2. In a separate saucepan, heat the chicken broth.

3. In a blender, add cooked chicken, garlic, soy sauce, green onion, ginger, powder, vinegar, and half of the chicken broth.

4. Blend until smooth, adding the remaining broth until desired consistency is reached.

5. Strain the puree to remove large pieces. Serve warm.

Lemon Salmon Puree

Serving: 2

Total time taken: 20 minutes

Ingredients

- 6 oz canned pink salmon
- 2 tablespoons Greek yogurt
- ½ teaspoon lemon juice
- ½ tablespoon fresh chives (chopped)
- 2 tablespoons shallots (chopped)
- Olive oil
- Salt

Directions

1. In a blender, add salmon, yogurt, lemon juice, chives, shallots, and salt.

2. Blend until smooth, adding water or olive oil to reach desired consistency.

3. Strain the puree to remove large pieces. Serve warm or at room temperature, as preferred.

Lemony Mustard Puree

Serving: 4

Total time taken: 20 minutes

Ingredients

- 8 oz boiled chicken breast (shredded)
- ¾ cup chicken broth
- 2 tablespoons Dijon mustard
- 2 tablespoons lemon juice
- 1 teaspoon brown sugar truvia
- Salt

Directions

1. In a medium sized pot, cover chicken with water and bring to a boil. Cook until done, about 15 minutes.

2. In a separate saucepan, heat the chicken broth.

3. In a blender, add cooked chicken, mustard, lemon juice, brown sugar, salt, and half of the chicken broth.

4. Blend until smooth, adding the remaining broth until desired consistency is reached.

5. Strain the puree to remove large pieces. Serve warm.

Worcestershire and Cream Puree

Serving: 4

Total time taken: 20 minutes

Ingredients

- 8 oz boiled chicken breast (shredded)
- 1 cup chicken broth
- 1 tablespoon Worcestershire sauce
- ½ cup fat-free half&half
- ½ cup skim milk
- Salt

Directions

1. In a medium sized pot, cover chicken with water and bring to a boil. Cook until done, about 15 minutes.

2. In a separate saucepan, heat the chicken broth.

3. In a blender, add cooked chicken, milk, half & half, Worcestershire sauce, salt, and half of the chicken broth.

4. Blend until smooth, adding the remaining broth until desired consistency is reached.

5. Strain the puree to remove large pieces. Serve warm.

Indian Curry Chicken Puree

Serving: 4

Total time taken: 20 minutes

Ingredients

- 8 oz boiled chicken breast (shredded)
- 1 cup chicken broth
- 2 tablespoons Greek yogurt
- ½ cup skim milk
- ½ cup tomatoes (chopped)
- ½ tablespoon curry powder
- 1 clove garlic
- Salt

Directions

1. In a medium sized pot, cover chicken with water and bring to a boil. Cook until done, about 15 minutes.

2. In a separate saucepan, heat the chicken broth.

3. In a blender, add cooked chicken, yogurt, milk, tomatoes, curry, salt, and half of the chicken broth.

4. Blend until smooth, adding the remaining broth until desired consistency is reached.

5. Strain the puree to remove large pieces. Serve warm.

Parmesan Tilapia Puree

Serving: 4

Total time taken: 20 minutes

Ingredients

- 8 oz steamed tilapia fillet (chopped
- ¾ cup chicken broth
- 1 tablespoon pesto
- 1 teaspoon lemon juice
- 2 tablespoons parmesan cheese
- ¼ cup chopped tomatoes
- Salt and pepper

Directions

1. In medium sized pot, bring a few inches of water to a boil. Add tilapia fillet to a steaming basket. Cover and steam until cooked, about 15 minutes.

2. In a separate saucepan, heat the chicken broth.

3. In a blender, add cooked tilapia, tomatoes, parmesan cheese, pesto, lemon juice, salt, pepper, and half of the chicken broth.

4. Blend until smooth, adding the remaining broth until desired consistency is reached.

5. Strain the puree to remove large pieces. Serve warm.

Crab Shallot Puree

Serving: 4

Total time taken: 20 minutes

Ingredients

- 1 6 oz can crab meat
- 1 cup chicken broth
- 2 tablespoons mayonnaise
- ½ teaspoon Old Bay seasoning
- 2 tablespoons shallots (chopped)

Directions

1. In a saucepan, heat the chicken broth.

2. In a blender, add crab meat, mayonnaise, seasoning, shallots, and half of the chicken broth.

3. Blend until smooth, adding the remaining broth until desired consistency is reached.

4. Strain the puree to remove large pieces. Serve warm.

Cauliflower and Cheese Mash

Serving: 6

Total time taken: 30 minutes

Ingredients

- 1 cauliflower head (finely chopped)
- 1 cup cheddar cheese (shredded)
- 1 cup sour cream
- 2 cloves garlic
- Salt and pepper, to taste

Directions

1. In a medium pot of boiling water, blanch cauliflower until soft, about 10-15 minutes. Drain.

2. In a blender, add blanched cauliflower, sour cream, cheese, garlic, salt, and pepper.

3. Blend until smooth, adding warm water to reach desired consistency.

4. Strain the puree to remove large pieces. Serve warm.

Creamy Lemon Shrimp Puree

Serving: 4

Total time taken: 20 minutes

Ingredients

- 8 oz frozen shrimp (chopped)
- ¼ cup sour cream
- ¼ cup parmesan cheese
- ¼ cup cream cheese
- 2 tablespoons lemon juice
- 1 clove garlic (minced)
- 2 tablespoons mayonnaise
- ¼ teaspoon red pepper flakes

Directions

1. In a pan, saute garlic, shrimp, lemon juice, and red pepper flakes for 2 minutes.

2. In a blender, add sauteed shrimp, cream cheese, sour cream, parmesan, and mayonnaise.

3. Blend until smooth, adding warm water until desired consistency is reached.

4. Strain the puree to remove large pieces. Serve warm.

Jalapeno Bean Puree

Serving: 4

Total time taken: 20 minutes

Ingredients

- 15 oz canned pinto beans
- 3 oz canned jalapeno peppers
- ¼ teaspoon paprika
- ¼ teaspoon onion powder
- ¼ teaspoon sugar
- 1 tablespoon white vinegar
- Salt

Directions

1. In a blender, add beans, jalapenos, vinegar, and spices.

2. Blend until smooth, adding warm water until desired consistency is reached.

3. Serve with tortilla chips as a side dip.

Gastric Sleeve Breakfast Recipes

Cinnamon Sugar Oatmeal Casserole

Serving: 8

Total time taken: 50 minutes

Ingredients

- 2 cups quick-cooking oats
- 1 cup buttermilk
- 2 eggs
- ½ cup unsweetened applesauce
- ⅓ cup craisins
- 2 tablespoons almonds (slivered)
- 1 ½ teaspoons cinnamon
- 1 teaspoon vanilla extract
- ⅓ cup splenda
- 1 ½ teaspoons baking powder
- ½ teaspoon salt

Directions

1. Preheat oven to 325 F. Coat a pie plate with cooking spray.

2. In a large bowl, combine oats, cinnamon, splenda, baking powder, and salt. Mix well.

3. In a separate bowl, beat together buttermilk, eggs, and applesauce. Pour into bowl with dry ingredients and combine until thoroughly mixed. Add in almonds and craisins.

4. Pour into a pie plate. Bake for 40-45 minutes.

5. Cool entirely before serving.

Vanilla Ricotta Muffins

Serving: 4

Total time taken: 40 minutes

Ingredients

- 2 cups ricotta cheese
- 3 teaspoons splenda
- 2 teaspoons vanilla extract
- 4 large eggs
- Berries (optional)

Directions

1. Preheat oven to 400 F.

2. Fill a muffin tin with tin liners. Coat with nonstick spray.

3. In a bowl, stir together all ingredients until smooth.

4. (Optional) If desired, add berries into the bowl and stir.

5. Pour into muffin cups.

6. Bake for 20-30 minutes, or until an inserted toothpick comes out clean.

Egg and Ham Breakfast Cups

Serving: 4

Total time taken: 40 minutes

Ingredients

- 6 eggs
- 6 slices deli ham
- 1 tablespoon cheddar cheese (shredded)
- Chives
- Salt and pepper, to taste

Directions

1. Preheat oven to 350 F.

2. Fill a muffin pan with tin liners. Coat with nonstick spray.

3. Line the muffin cups with ham slices. (If the edges stick up, that's fine). Bake for 10 minutes.

4. Break one egg into each cup. Sprinkle with salt and pepper. Bake for another 10 minutes.

5. Cook eggs to your liking. Remove from oven and top with cheese and chives. Serve warm.

Broccoli Mushroom Quiche

Serving: 4

Total time taken: 40 minutes

Ingredients

- 1 head of broccoli
- 3 oz Swiss cheese (low fat)
- ¼ cup skim milk
- 1 cup egg substitute
- ¼ cup half and half (fat-free)
- ½ cup canned mushrooms

Directions

1. Preheat oven to 400 F. Coat a pie plate with cooking spray.

2. In a pot, bring a few inches of water to a boil. Add broccoli to a steaming basket and steam. Chop broccoli to pieces sized as desired.

3. Add mushrooms and broccoli to pie plate.

4. In a bowl, mix half and half, skim milk, and egg substitute thoroughly. Pour over mushrooms and broccoli. Top with cheese.

5. Bake for 40 minutes. Serve warm.

Fruity Breakfast Popsicles

Serving: 4

Total time taken: 40 minutes

Ingredients

- 1 cup Greek yogurt
- ½ cup 1% milk
- ½ cup oats
- 1 cup mixed berries (or fruit of choice)

Directions

1. Mix yogurt and milk together, and divide mixture into popsicle molds.

2. Stir berries and oats into each mold.

3. Add a wooden stick into each mold. Put popsicle trays in freezer.

4. Freeze for a minimum of 4 hours before serving.

Whole Wheat Homemade Pretzels

Serving: 8

Total time taken: 50 minutes

Ingredients

- 2 ½ tablespoons active dry yeast
- 2 ½ cups white whole wheat flour
- 2 teaspoons baking soda
- 2 tablespoons agave or honey
- 2 tablespoons melted butter
- ½ teaspoon salt
- 1 cup warm water
- Coarse sea or pretzel salt (for topping)

Directions

1. In a stand mixer with a dough hook attachment, add all ingredients. Mix on medium speed. The dough should be sticky. Increase speed, kneading for 10 minutes.

2. Cover the bowl and let the dough rise for 30 minutes.

3. Preheat oven to 450 F. Divide dough into 8 pieces on a floured surface. Using your hands, roll out the dough lengthwise and twist it into a desired pretzel shape.

4. Bring a wide pot with a few inches of water to a boil. Whisk in baking soda until dissolved. Drop each pretzel into the boiling water until they float, usually 20 seconds. Scoop out with a slotted spoon.

5. Coat a nonstick baking sheet with cooking spray. Place pretzels on the sheet and top with pretzel salt to taste. Let the dough rest for 5-10 minutes.

6. Bake the pretzels for about 9 minutes. Switch pretzels to the broiler for 1-2 minutes, or until golden brown.

Spinach and Turkey Crustless Quiche

Serving: 8

Total time taken: 60 minutes

Ingredients

- Cooking spray
- 2 large eggs
- 2 large egg whites
- ½ cup all-purpose flour
- 1 teaspoon baking powder
- 4 oz. smoked turkey or ham (cubed)
- 1 clove garlic (minced)
- ½ cup onion (chopped)
- ⅛ teaspoon black pepper
- ¾ cup Swiss cheese (shredded), divided use
- ¼ cup extra sharp cheddar cheese (shredded)
- 1 cup cottage cheese
- ½ cup half & half
- 1 cup baby spinach leaves (fresh)

Directions

1. Preheat oven to 350 F.

2. In a nonstick skillet, sauté turkey, garlic, onion, and ground pepper over medium/high heat, until onions are tender or turkey is lightly browned. Set aside.

3. Coat a 9-inch pie plate with cooking spray. Apply ¼ cup of Swiss cheese on the bottom of the pie plate. Layer turkey and onion mixture on top.

4. Combine remaining ½ cup swiss cheese, cheddar cheese, spinach leaves, cottage cheese, half & half, and eggs into a large bowl. Whisk until it becomes a well-combined egg mixture.

5. In a separate bowl, mix flour and baking powder. Add to egg mixture. Fold together until well combined.

6. Layer the above mixture into pie plate. Bake for 45 minutes, or until knife comes out clean.

Cheesy Chili Egg Puff

Serving: 3

Total time taken: 45 minutes

Ingredients

- 1 can green chilies (chopped)
- 4 cups Monterey Jack cheese (chredded)
- 2 cups 4% cottage cheese
- 10 large eggs
- 1 teaspoon baking powder
- ½ cup all-purpose flour
- ½ teaspoon salt

Directions

1. Preheat oven to 350 F.

2. Beat the eggs in a large bowl on medium-high speed until eggs become light and creamy, or for about 3 minutes.

3. While beating, slowly sift baking powder, flour, and salt. Mix well.

4. Combine chilies and cheeses to the batter.

5. Pour the batter into a medium-sized, greased baking dish. Bake (uncovered) for 35-40 minutes, or until knife comes out clean. Cool for 5 minutes before serving.

Crustless Vegetable Quiche

Serving: 6

Total time taken: 60 minutes

Ingredients

- Olive oil
- Salt and Pepper
- 5 eggs
- ⅔ cup almond milk, unsweetened
- 4 oz. feta or goat cheese (crumbled)
- 1 cup green peas (frozen or fresh)
- 1 cup asparagus (sliced)
- 1 red bell pepper (diced)
- 3 green onions (sliced), optional
- 2 tablespoons fresh parsley (chopped)

Directions

1. Preheat oven to 350 F.

2. Heat olive oil in large skillet. Sauté peas, asparagus, bell pepper, and green onions over medium-high heat. Add salt and pepper. Cook until tender, about 5-6 minutes.

3. Put vegetables into a baking dish. Sprinkle goat cheese and parsley on top. Set aside.

4. In a separate bowl, combine the almond milk, eggs, and a pinch of salt and pepper. Whisk thoroughly. Pour over the vegetables.

5. Bake for 40-45 minutes, or until knife comes out clean. Cool for 20 minutes before serving

Greek Spinach and Feta Omelet

Serving: 1

Total time taken: 15 minutes

Ingredients

- 3 egg whites
- 6 cherry tomatoes (sliced)
- 2 tablespoons feta cheese (crumbled)
- ¼ cup spinach (chopped)
- Salt and pepper, to taste
- Cooking spray

Directions

1. Coat a skillet with cooking spray, and heat over medium heat.

2. Whisk egg whites, salt, and pepper until frothy.

3. Cook egg whites in skillet, about 1-2 minutes.

4. Place feta cheese, tomatoes, and spinach in the center of the egg. Continue to cook until egg edges curl up, about 2-3 minutes.

5. Fold the omelet in half. Cook until the cheese has melted, about 2-3 minutes. Serve immediately.

Cinnamon Pecan French Toast

Serving: 12

Total time taken: 60 minutes

Ingredients

- 2 cans cinnamon rolls (refrigerated)
- 6 eggs
- ¼ cup butter (melted)
- 2 teaspoons vanilla
- 2 teaspoons ground cinnamon
- 1 cup pecans (chopped)
- 1 cup maple syrup
- Powdered sugar
- ½ cup heavy whipping cream
- Icing (from cinnamon roll can)

Directions

1. Preheat oven to 375 F.

2. Coat 9" baking dish with melted butter.

3. Open the cans and separate the cinnamon rolls; there should be 16. Cut each roll into 8 pieces and put them in the baking dish. Set icing aside.

4. In medium bowl, beat the eggs. Whisk in the cinnamon, vanilla, and whipping cream until well mixed. Pour into the baking dish over the dough. Drizzle with maple syrup and top with chopped pecans.

5. Bake until the tops are golden brown, or for 20-25 minutes. Set aside to cool for 15 minutes.

6. Drizzle heated icing on top and serve immediately.

Chocolatey Zucchini Muffin

Serving: 12

Total time taken: 35 minutes

Ingredients

- 1 cup zucchini (shredded)
- ½ cup chocolate chips
- ¼ cup Greek yogurt or applesauce (unsweetened)
- ½ cup almond milk
- ⅓ cup cocoa powder (unsweetened)
- ⅓ cup honey
- 1 egg
- 1 egg white
- 1 teaspoon baking soda
- ¼ teaspoon salt
- 1 ¼ cup pastry flour or white flour (whole wheat)

Directions

1. Preheat oven to 350 F.

2. Remove excess water from shredded zucchini using paper towels.

3. Whisk together dry ingredients: cocoa powder, flour, salt, and baking soda. Set aside.

4. Whisk together honey, coconut oil, egg white, egg, and vanilla until smooth.

5. Add in applesauce (or yogurt), almond milk, and zucchini until well mixed.

6. Slowly mix in dry ingredients until well-combined. Stir in chocolate chips.

7. Line a standard muffin tray with cupcake liners. Evenly divide batter into liners.

8. Bake for about 22-25 minutes, or until an inserted toothpick comes out clean. Cool on wire rack before serving.

Lemony Poppy Seed Muffins

Serving: 12

Total time taken: 35 minutes

Ingredients

- 2 lemons (juiced and zested)
- 2 tablespoons poppy seeds
- 1 cup confectioners sugar
- ¾ cup all-purpose flour
- ¾ cup white sugar
- 2 ⅔ teaspoons baking powder
- 1 cup buttermilk
- ⅓ cup vegetable oil
- ⅓ cup sour cream
- ½ teaspoon salt
- 1 egg

Directions

1. Preheat oven to 350 F.

2. Mix white sugar, baking powder, flour, poppy seeds, lemon zest, and salt together in a large bowl.

3. In another bowl, beat together the sour cream, vegetable oil, buttermilk, and egg. Add to dry ingredients and stir until well combined.

4. Line a standard muffin tray with cupcake liners. Fill liners with batter until about ¾ full.

5. Bake for about 20 minutes, or until an inserted toothpick comes out clean. Place on wire rack to cool to room temperature.

6. Make a glaze by whisking lemon juice and confectioners' sugar until smooth. Drizzle over muffins and serve.

Soft Breakfast Whole Wheat Rolls

Serving: 24

Total time taken: 3 hours

Ingredients

- 4½ cups whole wheat flour
- 2 tablespoons active dry yeast
- 1 cup lukewarm milk
- ½ cup butter (softened)
- ½ cup warm water
- 3 eggs
- ¼ cup honey
- 1-½ teaspoons salt

Directions

1. Mix yeast and warm water in a glass. Dissolve and set aside to bloom.

2. In a stand mixer, whip the butter and honey using the paddle attachment until creamy.

3. Mix in the eggs thoroughly. Add the yeast and milk. Mix thoroughly.

4. Add in flour and salt. Switch to a dough hook attachment and knead until dough is no longer tacky, about 2-3 minutes. (More flour may be needed).

5. Cover the bowl and let the dough rise, usually for about one hour.

6. On a floured surface, knead the dough. Let it rest for 3 minutes. Roll the dough into 24 equal sized balls.

7. Arrange dough balls into a 13" baking dish. Cover and let rise, for about an hour.

8. Preheat oven to 350 F. Bake for 20-25 minutes, or until rolls are golden brown.

Gastric Sleeve Soup & Salads Recipes

Honey Glazed Salmon with Avocado Strawberry Salad

Serving: 4

Total time taken: 30 minutes

Ingredients

- 4 wild Atlantic salmon fillets
- 1 teaspoon liquid smoke
- 1 tablespoon honey
- 1 tablespoon lemon juice
- 2 tablespoons olive oil
- 6 cups lettuce mix
- 4 oz feta cheese or gorgonzola (crumbled)
- 1 red onion (thinly sliced)
- 1 avocado (cubed)
- 1 pint strawberries (sliced)
- ¼ cup toasted almonds (sliced)
  For the dressing:

- 2 tablespoons balsamic vinegar
- ¼ cup olive oil
- 1 teaspoon Dijon mustard
- 1 tablespoon honey
- ¼ teaspoon garlic powder
- Salt and pepper to taste

Directions

1. Preheat grill to medium-high heat.

2. Coat salmon fillets with olive oil. Grill salmon on grill, about 4-5 minutes per side.

3. Whisk together liquid smoke, honey, lemon juice, olive oil, and salt to make glaze. Brush glaze over each cooked salmon fillet. Set aside.

4. Whisk together balsamic vinegar, olive oil, mustard, honey, garlic powder, salt, and pepper to make dressing.

5. In 4 dinner plates, divide lettuce and top with cheese, red onion, avocado, strawberries, and almonds. Pour dressing over salads and top with salmon fillets.

Basil, Pepper, and Roasted Tomato Soup

Serving: 6

Total time taken: 1 hour 30 minutes

Ingredients

- 8 tomatoes (quartered)
- 1 yellow onion (quartered)
- 2 red peppers (quartered)
- 1 cup basil leaves (thinly sliced)
- 1 quart chicken broth
- 2 tablespoons red wine
- ¼ cup olive oil
- 1 teaspoon garlic powder
- 1 teaspoon dry thyme
- ¼ teaspoon red pepper flakes
- Salt and pepper, to taste

Directions

1. Preheat oven to 400 F.

2. Toss tomatoes, peppers, and onions with olive oil, salt, and pepper. Arrange on a baking sheet lined with parchment paper. Bake for 40 minutes.

3. Once vegetables cool completely, add to a blender with basil to make puree.

4. Over medium heat, pour the vegetable puree and red wine in a saucepan. Add garlic powder, thyme, red pepper flakes, salt, and pepper. Let it simmer for 2-3 minutes.

5. Add chicken broth and bring to a boil. Reduce to a low simmer, cover, and cook for 40 minutes.

6. Serve warm with crusty bread or grilled cheese.

Springy Chicken Salad

8.

Serving: 1

Total time taken: 20 minutes

Ingredients

- 1 ½ cups grilled chicken breasts (diced)
- ¼ cup diced celery
- ¼ cup craisins
- ½ cup grapes (sliced)
- 3 tablespoons light miracle whip

Directions

1. Preheat grill. Season chicken breasts as desired and grill until cooked, about 4 minutes per side. Dice the chicken breast into cubes. Cool completely.

2. In a large bowl, add chicken breast, craisins, grapes, celery, and miracle whip. Mix until all ingredients are coated evenly.

3. Serve as a salad on a bed of greens or on bread as a sandwich.

Balsamic Black Bean Salad

Serving: 1

Total time taken: 10 minutes

Ingredients

- 1 cup corn
- 2 cans black beans
- 2 tablespoons red onion (minced)
- 1 teaspoon garlic (minced
- ¼ cup fresh parsley (chopped)
- ¼ cup balsamic vinegar
- 1 teaspoon lemon juice
- 2 tablespoons olive oil
- 1 teaspoon honey
- Salt and pepper, to taste

Directions

1. In a large bowl, mix black beans, corn, onion, and parsley together.

2. In a separate bowl, whisk together balsamic vinegar, lemon juice, olive oil, honey, salt, and pepper. Pour over black bean salad.

3. Let the salad sit for 30 minutes, for flavors to blend.

4. Serve with pita chips, or over a bed of lettuce, as preferred.

Lentil and Ham Smoky Stew

Serving: 4-6

Total time taken: 1 hour 30 minutes

Ingredients

- 3 slices of bacon (thick-cut)
- ¾ cup lentils
- 4 cups chicken broth
- 1 carrot (diced in ¼" pieces)
- 1 stalk celery (diced in ¼" pieces)
- 1 yellow onion (diced)
- ¼ cup canned diced tomatoes
- 1 teaspoon garlic (minced)
- 1 teaspoon smoked paprika
- 1 tablespoon tomato paste
- Salt and pepper, to taste
- Sour cream (for garnish)

Directions

1. Heat skillet over medium-high heat. Cook bacon until crisp, 5-6 minutes. Drain excess oil with paper towels and chop into thick pieces.

2. In a Dutch oven pot, heat olive oil. Sauté garlic, onion, carrot, celery, paprika, and tomato paste over medium heat. Lower the heat to low.

3. Cover the pot and cook until vegetables soften, about 25 minutes, stirring occasionally.

4. Add broth, tomatoes, and lentils. Turn heat to high and bring to a boil.

5. Lower the heat and cover the pot. Simmer until lentils are tender, about 35-40 minutes, stirring occasionally. Add salt and pepper, to taste.

6. Using an immersion blender, puree the soup.

7. In warmed bowls, add soup for immediate serving. Garnish with bacon and sour cream.

Honey-Dressed Beet Salad

Serving: 3

Total time taken: 40 minutes

Ingredients

- 1 cup fresh spinach (chopped)
- 2 beets (sliced)
- 1 green apple (chopped)
- 2 spring onions (finely chopped)
- 2 tablespoons lime juice
- 3 tablespoons olive oil
- 1 tablespoon honey
- 1 tablespoon apple cider vinegar
- 1 teaspoon salt

Directions

1. In a deep pot, cover beets with water and cook until tender, for about 40 minutes. Remove skin and slice.

2. In a small bowl, add olive oil, honey, vinegar, lime juice, and salt. Mix thoroughly. Set aside for flavors to blend.

3. In a large bowl, add beets, spring onions, apple, and spinach. Mix well. Drizzle with dressing and mix to coat all ingredients.

4. Serve immediately.

Southwestern Style Creamy Chicken Soup

Serving: 8

Total time taken: 30 minutes

Ingredients

- 6 tablespoons all-purpose flour
- 1 cup chicken broth (low sodium)
- 3 cups whole milk
- 1 cup beer
- ½ cup white rice
- ½ teaspoon ground coriander
- 1 teaspoon chili powder
- 1 teaspoon ground cumin
- 1 tablespoon garlic (minced)
- 1 poblano Chile (diced)
- 1 red bell pepper (diced)
- ½ cup onion (diced)
- 2 cups cooked chicken (shredded)
- 3 cups pepperjack cheese (shredded)
- 2 tablespoons fresh cilantro (chopped)
- 8 sprigs cilantro (for garnish)
- Tortilla chips (for garnish)
- Lime slice (for garnish)

Directions

1. In a large pot, melt butter and add in coriander, chili powder, cumin, garlic, poblano, bell pepper, and onion. Sweat until peppers soften, about 5 minutes.

2. Stir in flour to coat vegetables, cooking for 2 minutes. Whisk in chicken broth, milk, and beer until smooth. Bring to a simmer.

3. Stir in rice. Simmer to until tender, about 15 minutes.

4. In a resealable bag, toss together cheese with some flour to coat. Stir in a handful at a time to the soup, melting completely until adding more. Add chicken and cilantro, cooking 3-5 minutes.

5. Divide soup into bowls and garnish with tortilla chips and lime. Serve warm.

Curry Coconut Chicken Salad

Serving: 2

Total time taken: 10 minutes

Ingredients

- 2 cooked chicken breasts (cubed)
- ¼ cup coconut milk
- ½ tablespoon vinegar
- 2 tablespoons mayonnaise
- ¾ teaspoon curry powder
- 2 teaspoons sugar
- 2 tablespoons almonds (slivered, toasted)
- 2 tablespoons sweetened coconut (shredded, toasted)
- 1 tablespoon cilantro (chopped)
- 2 green onions (chopped)
- 1 stalk celery (diced)
- Salt and pepper, to taste

Directions

1. Whisk together coconut milk, vinegar, mayonnaise, curry powder, sugar, salt, and pepper into a bowl until creamy.

2. Add chicken, onion, celery, and cilantro into the bowl. Coat ingredients with the sauce.

3. Divide into two bowls, topping with almonds and coconut. Serve with crackers or bread.

Teriyaki Chicken Blended Soup

Serving: 4

Total time taken: 20

Ingredients

- 8 oz boiled chicken breast (shredded)
- 1 cup chicken broth
- 2 tablespoons soy sauce
- 1 tablespoon brown sugar truvia
- 1 tablespoon fresh ginger (grated)
- 1 clove garlic

Directions

1. In a medium sized pot, cover chicken with water and bring to a boil. Cook until done, about 15 minutes.

2. In a separate saucepan, heat the chicken broth.

3. In a blender, add cooked chicken, soy sauce, brown sugar, ginger, garlic, and half of the chicken broth.

4. Blend until smooth, adding the remaining broth until desired consistency is reached.

5. Strain the puree to remove large pieces. Serve warm.

Grecian Black and White Bean Salad

Serving: 4-6

Total time taken: 20 minutes

Ingredients

- 3 oz feta cheese (crumbled)
- 15 oz. can of black beans
- 15 oz. can of white beans
- ½ cup cucumber (diced)
- ⅓ cup red onion (chopped)
- ⅓ cup fresh mint leaves (chopped)
  For the dressing:

- 2 tablespoons agave nectar
- 3 tablespoons lemon juice
- ¼ cup olive oil
- ½ teaspoon oregano
- ½ teaspoon celery seed
- ½ teaspoon garlic powder
- Salt and pepper, to taste

Directions

1. Whisk together dressing ingredients into a small bowl.

2. Add feta, beans, cucumber, onion, and mint in a bowl. Pour in dressing and toss to coat all ingredients.

3. Chill in refrigerator for at least one hour before serving.

Grilled Steak Bean Salad

Serving: 4-6

Total time taken: 30 minutes

Ingredients

- 1 pound flank steak
- 1 tablespoon Worchestershire sauce
- 3 tablespoons soy sauce
- ½ teaspoon steak seasoning
- 2 cups fresh green beans (1" pieces)
- ½ cup roasted red bell peppers (chopped)
- ¼ red onion (thinly sliced)
- 1 can black beans
- 1 can white beans
- Cooking spray
- ¼ cup feta cheese (crumpled, for garnish)
  For the dressing:

- 2 tablespoons olive oil
- 3 tablespoons red wine or balsamic vinegar
- ¼ teaspoon dry oregano
- ¼ teaspoon salt
- ¼ teaspoon pepper

Directions

1. Make marinade for steak with Worchestershire sauce, soy sauce, salt, and pepper. Rub in steak seasoning. Marinate steak in refrigerator for 20 minutes.

2. Preheat grill and coat with cooking spray. Grill flank steak for 8 minutes per side. Let steak rest for 10 minutes in tented foil. Cut in thin slices across grain. Set aside.

3. Steam green beans until tender but crisp, for about 5 minutes. Immediately cool under cold water.

4. To make dressing, whisk together all dressing ingredients.

5. In a large bowl, add steamed beans, black and white beans, red pepper, and onion. Drizzle with dressing and coat all ingredients.

6. Divide bean salad into plates and top with steak and feta to serve.

Cajun Style Creamy Soup

Serving: 4

Total time taken: 20 minutes

Ingredients

- 8 oz boiled chicken breast (shredded)
- ¾ cup chicken broth
- 1 tablespoon Cajun seasoning
- 1 clove garlic
- ¼ cup onion (chopped)
- Salt
- Cooking spray

Directions

1. In a medium sized pot, cover chicken with water and bring to a boil. Cook until done, about 15 minutes.

2. In a separate saucepan, heat the chicken broth.

3. In a saucepan over medium heat, saute the garlic and onion until fragrant.

4. In a blender, add cooked chicken, onion, garlic, seasoning, and half of the chicken broth.

5. Blend until smooth, adding the remaining broth until desired consistency is reached.

6. Strain the puree to remove large pieces. Serve warm.

Bean and Beefy Chili Soup

Serving: 8

Total time taken: 30 minutes

Ingredients

- 1 pound lean ground beef
- 2 cans cut tomatoes
- 1 can black peans
- 1 can pinto beans
- 1 can kidney beans
- ½ cup red bell pepper (chopped)
- ½ cup yellow bell pepper (chopped)
- 1 cup onion (chopped)
- 3 cloves garlic (minced)
- 1 teaspoon vegetable oil
- 1 ½ tablespoon chili powder
- 1 teaspoon oregano
- 1 teaspoon dried cumin
- 1 tablespoon brown sugar
- Salt and pepper, to taste

Directions

1. Heat oil over medium-high heat in a heavy bottom pan. Add beef, bell peppers, garlic, and onion. Cook until vegetables are tender and beef is browned.

2. Stir in brown sugar, tomatoes, beans, and spices. Bring to a boil.

3. Reduce heat and simmer for 30 minutes, or until chili has reached desired consistency.

4. Serve with grated cheese and sour cream.

Caesar Chicken and Pasta Salad

Serving: 10

Total time taken: 40 minutes

Ingredients

- 2 grilled chicken breasts (diced)
- 6 leaves Romaine lettuce (thinly sliced)
- 1 pound penne pasta, cooked
- ⅓ cup sour cream
- 1 teaspoon Worcestershire sauce
- 1 cup mayonnaise
- 2 tablespoons lemon juice
- 2 anchovies (finely minced)
- 1 clove garlic (pressed)
- 4 green onions (sliced)
- 1 ½ cups grape tomatoes
- ½ cup Parmesan cheese (finely shredded)
- 1 ½ cups crutons
- Salt and pepper, to taste

Directions

1. Whisk together mayonnaise, Parmesan cheees, Worcestershire sauce, sour cream, lemon juice, anchovies, garlic, salt, and pepper to make sauce.

2. Toss half of sauce with pasta and refrigerate for 30 minutes.

3. Toss remaining sauce with salad ingredients (lettuce, tomatoes, green onions, crutons).

4. Add chilled pasta and salad together and toss in a bowl. Refrigerate mixed salads together for 20 minutes to let flavors settle. Serve cold.

Bacon & Chicken Corn Chowder

Serving: 4

Total time taken: 40 minutes

ngredients

- 2 ½ cups rotisserie chicken (shredded)
- 3 strips bacon (roughly chopped)
- 3 ears white corn (kernels removed, cobs reserved)
- 2 sprigs thyme
- 1 onion (diced)
- 15 oz chicken broth
- 3 cups milk
- 3 tablespoons flour
- Salt and pepper, to taste

Directions

1. In a large pot, cook bacon over medium heat until browned, about 5 minutes. Add onions, cooking until translucent.

2. Add flour and stir constantly until golden, about 1 minute.

3. Slowly add chicken broth, whisking constantly to break clumps. Whisk in milk.

4. Add corn cobs and thyme to pot. Simmer and cook, stirring occasionally, for about 15 minutes, to infuse flavor. Remove cobs and thyme.

5. Add corn kernels and shredded chicken. Bring to a simmer.

6. Serve hot.

Beefy Vegetable Blended Stew

Serving: 4

Total time taken: 30 minutes

Ingredients

- 8 oz lean ground beef
- ¾ cup chicken broth
- ½ cup carrot (chopped)
- ½ cup onion (chopped)
- 1 clove garlic (minced)
- 1 tablespoon fresh thyme (chopped)
- Salt
- Cooking spray

Directions

1. Coat a medium saucepan with cooking spray. Over medium heat, saute the onion, garlic, and carrot until fragrant. Add and brown the ground beef.

2. Once meat is browned, add half of the chicken broth and herbs to the saucepan. Cover and simmer for 20 minutes.

3. In a blender, add all ingredients. Blend until smooth, adding remaining chicken broth to reach desired consistency.

4. Strain the puree to remove large pieces. Serve warm

Beef and Bacon Old-Fashioned Stew

Serving: 6

Total time taken: 4 hours 30 minutes

Ingredients

- 1 ½ pounds beef chuck roast
- 8 oz English or Canadian bacon (chopped)
- 1 quart beef broth
- 1 ½ cups red wine
- 4 Russet potatoes (chopped in 1" cubes)
- 4 carrots (chopped into ½" thick rounds)
- 1 cup pearl onions
- 1 tablespoon thyme leaves
- 1 tablespoon butter
- ½ teaspoon black pepper
- 1 teaspoon salt

Directions

1. Heat butter in stock pot. Add and brown bacon.

2. Season beef with salt and pepper. Add beef and brown on each side, about 3 minutes.

3. Add vegetables, stock, and wine. Over medium-high heat, bring to a boil.

4. Lower heat, cover the pot, and simmer until meat is tender, about 4-5 hours.

5. Remove and shred the meat. Return shredded meat to the pot, raising temperature to medium-high. Simmer uncovered until the liquid is reduced by ⅓ cup.

6. Serve with fresh thyme.

Autumnal Beef and Vegetable Soup

Serving: 6

Total time taken: 2 hours 25 minutes

Ingredients

- 2 pounds boneless beef chuck roast (cut in ½" cubes)
- 6 cups beef broth
- 3 cups green cabbage (chopped)
- 2 Yukon gold potatoes (diced)
- 1 onion (chopped)
- 6 cloves garlic (chopped)
- 4 carrots (diced)
- 1 cup corn kernels
- 1 cup peas
- 28 oz. canned diced tomato
- 2 tablespoons thyme or marjoram (chopped)
- 3 bay leaves
- 2 tablespoons olive oil

Directions

1. Over medium-high heat, heat olive oil in a large pot. Season beef with salt and pepper. Sauté beef until outside is no longer pink, about 4 minutes.

2. Add carrots, onion, garlic, bay leaves, and thyme. Sauté for 5 minutes.

3. Add diced tomatoes, beef broth, potatoes, and cabbage. Bring to a simmer. Partially cover pot and simmer until tender, about 50 minutes.

4. Add and stir peas and corn kernels. Simmer for 5 minutes. Add more stock if soup is too thick.

5. Add salt and pepper to taste.

Grilled Shrimp Grecian Salad

Serving: 6

Total time taken: 30 minutes

Ingredients

- 1 pound medium shrimp (peeled, deveined)
- 4 oz. feta cheese (crumpled)
- 1 tomato (chopped)
- 1 cucumber (halved and sliced)
- 2 cups spinach leaves
- 6 cups romaine lettuce (chopped)
- ¾ cups Italian dressing, divided use

Directions

1. Marinate shrimp in ¼ cup Italian dressing for 30 minutes.

2. Grill or broil until fully cooked, turning shrimp once.

3. Toss shrimp with remaining ingredients in a large serving bowl. Serve immediately.

Blended Cauliflower and Broccoli Soup

Serving: 2

Total time taken: 20 minutes

Ingredients

- 2 cups cauliflower (chopped)
- 2 cups broccoli (chopped)
- ½ cup skim milk
- 1 tablespoon olive oil
- 1 teaspoon dry mint
- 1 tablespoon parsley (chopped)
- ½ teaspoon italian seasoning
- ½ teaspoon ground cumin
- Salt

Directions

1. In a medium pot, add cauliflower and cover with water. Bring water to a boil and cook for 15 minutes. Drain and set aside.

2. In a blender, add broccoli, cooked cauliflower, milk, salt, cumin, parsley, mint, and seasoning.

3. Blend until smooth, gradually adding olive oil to reach desired consistency.

4. Serve with fresh celery and carrots.

Traditional Minestrone Soup

Serving: 4

Total time taken: 45 minutes

Ingredients

- 5 oz. spaghetti
- 2 potatoes (diced)
- 1 onion (chopped)
- 4 celery stalks (chopped)
- 2 cloves garlic (minced)
- 3 carrots (chopped)
- ½ head cabbage (shredded)
- 2 tablespoons tomato purée
- 3 ½ cups vegetable broth
- 14 oz. can butter
- 14 oz. can chopped tomato
- 1 tablespoon olive oil
- Crusty bread, for serving

Directions

1. Heat oil in a pan. Add vegetables, garlic, and potatoes. Cook over high heat until softened, about 5 minutes.

2. Stir in chopped tomatoes, tomato purée, and vegetable broth. Bring to a boil, and then lower the heat. Cover and simmer for 10 minutes.

3. Add beans and pasta. Cook for 10 minutes. Add cabbage at the end, cooking until wilted.

4. Add salt and pepper to taste. Serve with crusty bread.

Orange Minty Salmon Salad

Serving: 2

Total time taken: 15 minutes

Ingredients

- 8 oz smoked salmon (sliced)
- 1 large tomato (chopped)
- 2 cups iceberg lettuce (chopped)
- 2 cucumbers (sliced)
- ¼ cup sweet corn
- 4 tablespoon orange juice
  For dressing:

- 1 ¼ cup yogurt
- 2 garlic cloves (crushed)
- 1 tablespoon fresh mint (chopped)
- 1 tablespoon sesame seeds

Directions

1. In a bowl, whisk together yogurt, garlic, mint, and sesame seeds.

2. In a larger bowl, combine lettuce, cucumbers, tomatoes, and corn. Top wtih salmon and drizzle with orange juice.

3. Pour dressing over salad, tossing well to combine flavors. Serve cold.

Orange Seafood Salad

Serving: 3

Total time taken: 35 minutes

Ingredients

- 1 cup frozen seafood of preference
- 5 tablespoons olive oil
- 2 cups lettuce
- 1 cucumber (sliced)
- 1 onion (finely chopped)
- ½ red bell pepper (sliced)
- 3 garlic cloves (crushed)
- ¼ cup orange juice
- Salt, to taste

Directions

1. In a skillet over medium-high heat, heat 3 tablespoons of olive oil. Saute onion and garlic for about 5 minutes.

2. Add frozen seafood of choice and reduce heat to medium. Cover and cook for 15 minutes. Set aside to cool.

3. In a large bowl, combine lettuce, cucumber and bell pepper in a bowl. Top with a dressing made of orange juice, remaining olive oil, and salt.

4. Top with cooked seafood and serve immediately.

Smoked Turkey and Arugula Salad

Serving: 4

Total time taken: 30 minutes

Ingredients

- 8 oz smoked turkey breast (cubed)
- 4 oz arugula
- 8 oz lettuce
- 2 oranges (peeled, sliced)
  For dressing:

- ¼ cup olive oil
- 1 teaspoon apple cider vinegar
- 3 tablespoons lemon juice
- ¼ cup Greek yogurt

Directions

1. In a large bowl, add lettuce, arugula, oranges, and turkey breast. Mix well to combine and set aside.

2. In a separate bowl, whisk together yogurt, lemon juice, olive oil, and apple cider vinegar.

3. Drizzle dressing over salad and serve.

Gastric Sleeve Lunch & Dinner Recipes

Lemon Tomato Couscous

Serving: 4

Total time taken: 25 minutse

Ingredients

- 5 oz couscous
- 1 cup vegetable broth
- 3 tablespoons olive oil
- 3 tablespoons lemon juice
- 3 tablespoons tomato sauce
- 1 onion (chopped)
- ½ cucumber (sliced)
- ½ carrot (sliced)
- ½ cup fresh parsley (chopped)
- Salt

Directions

1. In a saucepan, bring vegetable broth to a boil. Slowly add in couscous, stirring constantly. Cover and let sit for 10 minutes, until couscous absorbs all liquid. Set aside and occasionally fluff with a fork.

2. In a skillet, heat olive oil and tomato sauce over medium heat. Add onions and saute until translucent. Set aside to cool.

3. In a large bowl, add couscous, tomato onion sauce, lemon juice, parsley, and salt. Mix until well coated with the sauce.

4. Serve with carrot and cucumber slices.

Spring Veggie and Chicken Pasta

Serving: 6

Total time taken: 30 minutes

Ingredients

- 2 cups chicken breast (cooked, chopped)
- 3 cups penne pasta
- 1 cup broccoli florets
- ½ cup frozen corn
- ½ cup frozen peas
- 1 onion (diced)
- 1 tablespoon garlic (crushed)
- 1 red capsicum (diced)
- 1 teaspoon chicken stock powder
- 1 tablespoon dried parsley
- 1 cup reduced fat cheese (grated)
- 1 cup thickened cream
- Green onion (sliced)
- Fresh cilantro
- Peanuts (chopped)
- Salt and pepper, to taste
- Cooking spray

Directions

1. Cook pasta according to package directions. Set aside.

2. Coat a large frying pan with cooking spray. Over medium heat, sauté garlic and onion. Add peas, corn, broccoli, and capsicum. Cook until vegetables are tender but crisp.

3. Add cooked chicken to pan. Heat thoroughly. Add cream, chicken stock powder, parsley, salt, and pepper. Coat vegetables well with sauce. Then, stir in the cheese until melted.

4. Toss pasta into the skillet to combine. Coat pasta well with sauce.

5. Serve, garnished with chopped nuts, cilantro, and green onion.

Broccoli and Cauliflower Tuna Casserole

Serving: 6

Total time taken: 30 minutes

Ingredients

- 2 cans tuna
- 3 cups cauliflower
- 5 cups broccoli
- ¾ cups mayonnaise
- 8 oz cream cheese
- 2 cups cheddar cheese (shredded)
- 1 onion (chopped)
- 1 tablespoon Italian seasoning
- 1 teaspoon garlic powder
- ½ teaspoon celery seed powder
- ½ teaspoon red pepper flakes
- Salt and pepper, to taste

Directions

1. Preheat oven to 350 F.

2. In a medium bowl, mix tuna, cream cheese, mayonnaise, onion, and seasonings. Mix until well combined.

3. In a rectangular baking dish, layer broccoli and cauliflower. Spoon tuna mixture in another, even layer. Top with a layer of shredded cheese.

4. Bake for 30 minutes, or until the cheese is golden and bubbly. Serve warm.

Hungarian Paprika Chicken

Serving: 6

Total time taken: 2 hours

Ingredients

- 1 broiler chicken (4-5 pounds, cooked, cut in pieces)
- 2 tablespoons paprika
- 1 onion (chopped)
- ¼ cup butter (cubed)
- 1 cup sour cream
- 2 tablespoons cornstarch
- Salt and pepper, to taste
- 1 ½ cups water

Directions

1. Preheat oven to 350 F.

2. In a large skillet over medium-high heat, heat butter. Cook onion until tender.

3. Rub chicken with salt, pepper, and paprika. Place in a baking dish with water. Top with onions.

4. Bake for about 1- 1 ½ hours, or until the chicken is completely cooked.

5. In a separate bowl, mix cold water and cornstarch. Add juices from the cooked baking dish and the cornstarch mixture into the skillet the onions were cooked in. Bring the mixture to a boil. Cook and stir until thickened, for about 1-2 minutes.

6. Serve the baked chicken topped with sauce.

Chicken Veggie Asian Stir Fry

Serving: 6

Total time taken: 30 minutes

Ingredients

- 1 pound boneless, skinless chicken breast (sliced small)
- 3 cups brown rice (cooked)
- 1 tablespoon corn starch
- 1 tablespoon brown sugar
- 1 cup chicken broth
- ½ cup soy sauce
- ½ cup pineapple juice
- ½ zucchini (sliced in rounds and quartered)
- ½ cup broccoli florets
- ½ red bell pepper (sliced)
- 1 carrot (thinly sliced)
- ½ red onion (sliced)
- 2 tablespoons cilantro (chopped)
- 4-5 sugar snap peas
- ¼ cup toasted cashew
- 2 cloves garlic (minced)
- Green onion (thinly sliced, for garnish)
- 1 tablespoon fresh ginger (finely grated)
- 2 tablespoons vegetable oil

Directions

1. Marinate chicken with soy sauce and cornstarch.

2. In a large skillet over medium-high heat, heat 1 tablespoon of vegetable oil. Stir fry zucchini, snap peas, bell pepper, broccoli, ginger, carrot, onion, and garlic for 2-3 minutes.

3. Add chicken broth and cover until vegetables are tender, about 4-5 minutes.

4. In another frying pan, heat 1 tablespoon vegetable oil and cook chicken thoroughly.

5. Add stir fried vegetables, cilantro, and pineapple juice to the pan with cooked chicken.

6. Before serving, mix in cashews and cooked rice. Heat all together. Garnish with green onion.

Easy Chicken Parmesan

Serving: 6

Total time taken: 35 minutes

Ingredients

- 2 pounds chicken cutlets (pounded thin)
- 1 jar spaghetti sauce (low sodium)
- 8 oz part-skim mozzarella cheese (shredded)
- ¾ cup Parmesan cheese (grated)
- 2 eggs
- ¾ cup flour
- 1 ¾ cups Italian breadcrumbs
- ½ cup vegetable oil
- Salt and pepper, to taste

Directions

1. Preheat oven to 375 F.

2. In a bowl, beat together eggs and 2 tablespoons of water.

3. Set up 3 shallow dishes: 1 with flour + salt + pepper ; 1 with bread crumbs ; 1 with the eggs.

4. Dip chicken in flour. Shake off excess. Dip chicken in eggs. Drain excess. Dip in breadcrumbs. Coat chicken thoroughly.

5. In a large skillet, heat vegetable oil over medium-high heat. Add breaded chicken and cook until golden, about 2 minutes per side.

6. In a 13" baking pan, pour half of spaghetti sauce. Add one layer of chicken. Cover with half of mozzarella and Parmesan. Layer with leftover chicken, sauce, and cheeses.

7. Bake for about 20 minutes, or until cheese is bubbling. Serve warm.

Kale, Butternut Squash, and Sausage Pasta

Serving: 8

Total time taken: 1 hour

Ingredients

- 6 links Italian sausage (spicy or sweet)
- 4 cups kale (roughly chopped)
- 1 cup butternut squash (diced)
- 3 cloves garlic (grated)
- ¼ cup parsley (minced)
- 1 pound whole wheat pasta (orecchiette)
- ½ cup Parmigiano-Reggiano (grated)
- ¼ cup olive oil (divided)
- Salt and pepper, to taste

Directions

1. Preheat oven to 400 F.

2. Line a baking sheet with foil. Coat butternut squash with olive oil, salt, and pepper. Arrange onto a single layer on the baking sheet. Roast until golden brown, about 25-30 minutes. Toss once, halfway through.

3. Prepare orecchiette pasta according to package instructions. Set aside 1 cup of cooked pasta liquid. Set cooked pasta aside.

4. In a deep pan over medium-high heat, heat 1 tablespoon of olive oil. Remove sausage from casings and add to pan. Begin browning the meat.

5. Add grated garlic when sausage is halfway cooked. Continue cooking until thoroughly cooked, about 7-9 minutes. Deglaze pan with cooked pasta liquid.

6. Stir kale, 2 tablespoons of olive oil, salt, and pepper into sausage pan. Wait 2-3 minutes, until kale is bright green.

7. Toss in cooked pasta, roasted butternut squash, parsley, and Parmigiano-Reggiano.

8. Serve, topped with Parmigiano-Reggiano and parsley as preferred.

Lemon Juice Salmon With Quinoa

Serving: 2

Total time taken: 30 minutes

Ingredients

- 2 8-ounce boneless salmon fillets
- 14 cherry tomatoes (halved)
- 10 white button mushrooms (thinly sliced)
- 8-10 asparagus spears
- 1 lemon
- 2 tablespoon dill (roughly chopped)
- 2 cloves garlic (minced)
- 2 teaspoons olive oil
- 2 teaspoons capers (optional)

Directions

1. Preheat oven to 350 F.

2. On a large piece of parchment paper, layer minced garlic. Place layer of asparagus on top of garlic. Arrange a salmon fillet on top of the asparagus. Place the mushrooms and cherry tomatoes around the salmon.

3. Drizzle with lemon juice and olive oil. Season with salt, pepper, dill, and capers.

4. Fold paper up above the ingredients, careful to maintain the layered arrangement. Tightly seal by folding the edges several times.

5. Bake for 20-25 minutes, or until salmon is flaky.

6. Serve with rice, pasta, or quinoa.

Baja Mango Salsa and Fish Tacos

Serving: 4

Total time taken: 20 minutes

Ingredients

- 1 pound cod fillets
- 2 mangos (chopped)
- 1 tablespoon lime juice
- 1 tablespoon cilantro (chopped)
- ¼ cup red bell pepper (minced)
- 2 green onions (sliced)
- 1 jalapeno pepper
- ½ teaspoon Mexican oregano
- ½ teaspoon ground cumin
- ½ teaspoon garlic salt
- 1 teaspoon chili powder
- 8 corn tortillas
- 2 cups cabbage (shredded)
- ½ cup cotija cheese (crumbled)

Directions

1. Preheat oven to 425 F.

2. Rub cod with dry seasonings (oregano, cumin, garlic salt, chili powder).

3. Place cod on parchment paper. Take edges of paper and fold twice, tucking underneath the fish. Bake for 15-18 minutes. Open packets carefully to let steam escape.

4. In a bowl, stir bell pepper, mango, cilantro, onions, jalapeno, and lime juice. Set aside.

5. To serve, top corn tortillas with cod, mango salsa, cabbage, and cheese.

Spring Chicken and Veggie Soup

Serving: 4

Total time taken: 75 minutes

Ingredients

- 4 boneless chicken thighs
- 8 oz chicken stock
- 4 oz tomato paste
- 1 lb roasted tomatoes (diced)
- 2 cloves garlic (crushed)
- 1 onion (finely chopped)
- 3 carrots (chopped)
- 3 stalks celery (chopped)
- 2 chili peppers (finely chopped)
- 4 oz mushrooms
- 1 teaspoon dried basil
- 2 tablespoons olive oil
- Sour cream
- Salt and pepper, to taste

Directions

1. In a skillet over medium-high heat, heat olive oil. Saute carrots, onions, and celery for about 10 minutes.

2. In a deep pot, transfer cooked carrots, onions, and celery. Add mushrooms, garlic, basil, tomato paste, salt, and pepper. Coat vegetables well with tomato sauce.

3. Add chicken, chicken stock, and tomatoes into the pot. Lower heat and cook for an hour.

4. Serve warm and top with sour cream.

Potatoes and Swiss Chard

Serving: 3

Total time taken: 60 minutes

Ingredients

- 2 potatoes (finely chopped)
- 1 lb swiss chard (torn)
- 2 cloves garlic (finely chopped)
- 1 onion (chopped)
- 3 tablespoons olive oil
- Salt and pepper, to taste

Directions

1. In a large pot, cover swiss chard with water and bring to a boil. Cook until tender, about 3 minutes. Drain and set aside.

2. In a large skillet over medium-high heat, heat olive oil. Saute garlic and onions for about 3 minutes.

3. Add potatoes and 1 cup of water to skillet and bring to a boil. Reduce heat and cook for 15 minutes.

4. Add swiss chard to skillet, seasoning with salt and pepper to taste. Cook for 2 minutes.

5. Serve immediately.

Eggs in Avocado Shells

Serving: 4

Total time taken: 35 minutes

Ingredients

- 6 eggs
- 2 avocados (halved)
- 4 tablespoons Greek yogurt
- 3 tablespoons olive oil
- 1 tomato (finely chopped)
- 1 tablespoon rosemary (finely chopped)
- 2 tablespoons parsley (finely chopped)
- Salt and pepper, to taste

Directions

1. Preheat oven to 350 F.

2. Scrape out flesh from avocado shells and save for another use.

3. In a bowl, whisk together tomatoes, eggs, rosemary, parsley, salt, and pepper. Spoon into avocado shells.

4. Fill avocado shells with eggs mixture. Place on a greased baking sheet. Bake for 15 minutes. Let cool for 5 minutes.

5. Top with yogurt to serve.

Peanut Apple Chicken

Serving: 2

Total time taken: 35 minutes

Ingredients

- 2½ lbs chicken (cubed)
- ¼ cup mustard
- 15 oz unsweetened applesauce
- 1 cup powdered peanuts
- ⅛ cup brown sugar splenda
- Salt and pepper, to taste

Directions

1. In a skillet over medium heat, saute chicken until nearly done, about 12 minutes.

2. Add brown sugar, mustard, applesauce, and powdered peanuts. Stir together so chicken is well-coated with sauce.

3. Simmer until chicken is thoroughly cooked, about 5 minutes.

4. Serve warm, suggested with rice or salad.

Rice and Meat Stuffed Peppers

Serving: 4

Total time taken: 6 hours

Ingredients

- 4 bell peppers
- 1½ lbs lean ground beef
- 1½ cups brown rice
- 1 cup onion (chopped)
- 1 egg
- 2 cups tomato sauce
- 1 teaspoon garlic powder
- Salt and pepper, to taste

Directions

1. Cut peppers in half and remove the cores.

2. In a bowl, add ground beef, rice, onion, whisked egg, garlic powder, 1 cup of tomato sauce, salt, and pepper. Mix well.

3. Stuff the peppers with the mixture. Place in a slow cooker with the remaining cup of tomato sauce.

4. Cover and set to low. Cook until thoroughly ready, about 6 hours.

Pepper Pork Chops

Serving: 4

Total time taken: 20 minutes

Ingredients

- 4 - 3oz pork chops
- 1½ cups chicken broth
- 2 tablespoons corn starch
- 2 tablespoons olive oil
- ½ onion (sliced thin)
- ½ yellow bell pepper (sliced)
- ½ red bell pepper (sliced)
- ½ green bell pepper (sliced)
- ½ cup water

Directions

1. In a skillet over medium heat, saute pork in olive oil until both sides are browned. Remove from pan and set aside.

2. Add onion and peppers to the skillet. Saute until they are caramelized.

3. Add pork in the skillet and pour in the chicken broth. Cook until pork is no longer pink, about 15 minutes. Remove from the pan.

4. Dissolve corn starch into cold water and add to pan. Let the sauce thicken. Season with salt and pepper to taste.

5. Top the pork chops with pepper sauce. Serve with choice of side.

Rosemary Avocado Eggs

Serving: 6

Total time taken: 20 minutes

Ingredients

- 6 eggs
- 3 avocados (halved)
- 1 tomato (finely chopped)
- 2 teaspoons dried rosemary
- 3 tablespoons olive oil
- Salt and pepper, to taste

Directions

1. Preheat oven to 350 F.

2. Boil 6 eggs to preferred liking.

3. Cut avocados in half. Remove pits and flesh.

4. Stuff each avocado shell with a boiled egg and chopped tomatoes. Top with rosemary, salt, and pepper.

5. On a small, greased baking pan, arrange avocado shells tightly. Bake for about 20 minutes.

6. Let cool before serving.

Egg Whites and Sweet Potatoes

Serving: 4

Total time taken: 40 minutes

Ingredients

- 6 egg whites
- 4 sweet potatoes
- 2 onions (finely chopped)
- 4 tablespoons olive oil
- 1 tablespoon ground garlic
- Salt and pepper, to taste

Directions

1. Preheat oven to 350 F.

2. Coat a medium-sized baking sheet with olive oil. Spread peeled sweet potatoes on the sheet and bake for 20 minutes. Let potatoes cool on the side.

3. Cut sweet potatoes into thick slices and add in a bowl. Add egg whites, olive oil, chopped onions, garlic, salt, and pepper. Mix well.

4. Lower oven temperature to 200 F. Spread the sweet potato mixture onto a baking sheet and bake for 15-20 minutes.

5. Cool before serving.

BBQ Seasoned Chicken Thighs

Serving: 6

Total time taken: 40 minutes

Ingredients

- 2 lbs chicken thighs
- 2 tablespoons olive oil
- 2 cups chicken broth
- 2 onions (chopped)
- 1 red onion (chopped)
- 1 chili pepper
- ¼ cup unsweetened orange juice
- 1 teaspoon orange extract
- 1 teaspoon BBQ seasoning mix

Directions

1. Preheat oven to 350 F.

2. In a large saucepan over medium heat, saute onions in olive oil until golden.

3. Blend orange juice, orange extract, and chili pepper in a food processor for 30 seconds. Add to saucepan. Reduce heat.

4. Rub the chicken thighs with BBQ seasoning. Add into the saucepan.

5. Add chicken broth to saucepan and bring to a boil. Cook until water evaporates.

6. Place chicken in a large baking dish. Bake for 15 minutes for a golden, crispy skin.

Quinoa Coconut Thai Bowl

Serving: 4

Total time taken: 60 minutes

Ingredients

- 2 cups quinoa
- ¼ cup peanut butter
- 1 can coconut milk
- 1 tablespoon garlic (minced)
- 2 carrots (diced)
- 1 sweet potato (diced)
- 2 tablespoons olive oil
- ½ cup water
- 2 tablespoons cilantro (finely chopped)
- 2 tablespoons peanuts (crushed)
- Salt and pepper, to taste

For the Cabbage Slaw:

- 1 cup purple cabbage (finely chopped)
- 1 red pepper (diced)
- 1 cup edamame
- 1 lime (juiced)
- 1/4 teaspoon dried orange peel
- 1/4 teaspoon ginger powder
- 1/4 teaspoon garlic powder
- tablespoon maple syrup
- 2 tablespoons olive oil
- 1 tablespoon tamari (or soy sauce)

Directions

1. Preheat oven to 400 F.
2. In a medium-sized pot, bring quinoa, coconut milk, and water to a boil. Reduce heat and cover. Cook until all liquid has been absorbed, about 10 minutes. Fluff with fork and season with salt and pepper to taste.
3. Toss and coat diced vegetables with olive oil, garlic, salt, and pepper. Place vegetables on a large baking sheet and bake until tender, about 25-30 minutes.
4. In a large bowl, add endamame, red pepper, and cabbage. Separately mix remaining cabbage slaw ingredients together, and then toss to coat.
5. Assemble the bowl: layer coconut quinoa, roasted vegetables, and cabbage slaw. Sprinkle peanuts and cilantro. Mix peanut butter with olive oil for a drizzle.

Mongolian Broccoli Beef

Serving: 6

Total time taken: 30 minutes

Ingredients

- 1 lb. beef flank steak (thin cut)
- 1 sweet red pepper (cut in 1" pieces)
- 2 carrots (cut in ½" cubes)
- 3 cups broccoli florets
- 1 onion (thinly sliced)
- 3 garlic cloves (minced)
- 1 teaspoon fresh ginger (minced)
- 3 tablespoons olive oil, divided
- ½ cup soy sauce
- ¼ cup corn starch
- ½ cup soy sauce
- ½ cup coconut or brown sugar
- ¼ cup sliced green onion
- Salt and pepper to taste
- Hot rice for serving

Directions

1. In a large skillet, heat one tablespoon of olive oil. Sauté the ginger, onion, broccoli, carrots, pepper, and garlic until nearly tender, about 8-10 minutes. Set aside.

2. Coat beef cuts in cornstarch and let it sit for 10 minutes. Heat remaining oil in skillet over medium-high heat. Sauté beef cuts until browned.

3. Reduce heat and stir in soy sauce.

4. Mix remaining cornstarch and water together, adding it to the beef. Stir well. Add sugar and bring to a simmer.

5. Once thickened, add sautéed vegetables to the beef, making a stir fry. Add salt and pepper to taste. Garnish with green onions.

BBQ Sauce Italian Meatballs

Serving: 18

Total time taken: 1 hour 30 minutes

Ingredients

- ¾ pound ground beef
- ¾ pound ground turkey
- 1 egg white (lightly beaten)
- ¾ cup graham cracker crumbs
- 2 teaspoons prepared mustard
- 3 tablespoons milk

For the Sauce:

- 1 cup BBQ sauce
- 6 oz frozen orange juice concentrate (thawed)
- ¼ cup water

Directions

1. Preheat oven to 375 F.

2. Whisk together the graham cracker crumbs, milk, mustard, egg white, and salt in a large bowl.

3. Add ground beef and turkey, mixing until well combined.

4. Roll the mixture into 1 ½" balls. Arrange them on a greased baking sheet.

5. Bake until the meat is no longer pink, about 20 minutes. Transfer meatballs onto a deeper baking dish.

6. Combine sauce ingredients and mix well. Pour over meatballs.

7. Lower the oven temperature to 350 F. Cover the dish with aluminum foil. Bake for 1 hour.

Pears, Apples & Pork Chops

Serving: 2

Total time taken: 30 minutes

Ingredients

- 4 boneless pork chops
- 3 tablespoons brown sugar
- 2 teaspoons cinnamon
- 1 pear (chopped)
- 1 apple (chopped)
- 3 tablespoons butter
- 2-3 tablespoons bourbon
- 1 ½ teaspoons thyme

Directions

1. In a nonstick skillet over medium-low heat, melt butter. Add cinnamon and brown sugar, cooking until melted.

2. Add and coat the apples in the skillet. Cook until softened, about 3 minutes. Add in the pears and cook for 3 minutes.

3. Turn the fire high and remove the pan from heat. Pour in the bourbon, tipping the pan to the flame until it ignites. (*Only perform this step if you are comfortable with handling fire. You can also cook off the bourbon without the fire.*) Cook, about 2 or 3 minutes. Set aside and add thyme.

4. In a cast iron pan, heat oil over medium-high heat. Apply salt and pepper to porkchops, to taste. Cook each side until medium, about 3 minutes per side.

5. Top porkchops with cooked fruits to serve.

Fiesta Chipotle Tacos

Serving: 4

Total time taken: 20

Ingredients

- 1 pound pork tenderloin
- 2 teaspoons chili in adobo sauce (chopped)
- 2 teaspoons garlic (minced)
- 1 cup shallots (thinly sliced)
- 1 ½ lime (grated rind)
- 1 tablespoon lime juice
- 2 teaspoons oregano
- 1 teaspoon brown sugar
- ¼ teaspoon salt
- 2 teaspoons olive oil
- Cooking spray
- Chopped cilantro
- 8x (6") corn tortillas
- ¼ cup sour cream

Directions

1. Cut pork into strips. Marinate in lime juice, garlic, chili, brown sugar, oregano, salt.

2. Coat nonstick skillet in cooking spray over medium heat. Sauté shallots until tender, about 4 minutes. Set aside.

3. Sauté pork until no longer pink, about 3 minutes. Add shallots to the skillet and heat together.

4. For serving: warm up tortillas (according to package directions). Layer pork, sour cream, and cilantro on each tortilla.

Vegetable and Steak Brochettes

Serving: 10

Total time taken: 25 minutes

Ingredients

- 2 ½ lbs. Sirloin steak (cut in 1 ¼ " pieces)
- 1 onion (cut in wedges)
- 2 zucchini (cut in 1" slices)
- 24 fresh mushrooms
- 24 cherry tomatoes
- 1 large bell pepper (cut in 1 ½ " cubes)
- Cooked rice
  For the Marinade:

- ¼ cup lemon juice
- ¼ cup soy sauce
- ¼ cup canola oil
- 2 cloves garlic (minced)
- 2 cloves (whole)
- ¼ cup brown sugar
- A pinch of dried basil

Directions

1. Whisk marinade ingredients in a large bowl. Set aside.

2. Arrange vegetables and meat on bamboo skewers. Cover with marinade and refrigerate overnight, turning kebabs throughout.

3. Cook kebabs on the grill, thoroughness to taste.

4. Suggested serving is with rice.

Beef and Zucchini Lasagna

Serving: 4

Total time taken: 1 hour 30 minutes

Ingredients

- ½ pound ground beef
- 1 egg
- ¾ cup cottage cheese
- ½ cup mozzarella cheese (shredded)
- 1 can tomato paste
- 2 ½ cups zucchini (¼" lengthwise slices)
- ¼ cup onion (chopped)
- 2 small tomatoes (chopped)
- 1 clove garlic (minced)
- ½ teaspoon dried basil
- ½ teaspoon dried oregano
- ¼ teaspoon dried thyme
- 1 teaspoon flour
- ¼ cup water
- Salt and pepper to taste

Directions

1. Preheat oven to 375 F.

2. In a nonstick skillet, cook zucchini until tender and set aside.

3. On medium-high heat, fry the meat and onions until cooked.

4. Add tomatoes, tomato paste, oregano, thyme, basil, garlic, and water. Simmer uncovered until sauce is reduced.

5. In a separate bowl, beat eggs, cottage cheese, mozzarella cheese, and flour.

6. Layer zucchini, meat, and cheese mixtures.

7. Bake uncovered for 30 minutes.

8. Cover lasagna with the cheese left. Set in the broiler until cheese is golden, about 5 minutes.

9. Cool 10 minutes before serving.

Vegetables and Grilled Steak

Serving: 4

Total time taken: 55 minutes

Ingredients

- 1 lb veal steak (1" thick)
- 3 tablespoons olive oil
- 1 green bell pepper (sliced)
- 1 red bell pepper (sliced)
- Salt and pepper, to taste

Directions

1. Heat olive oil in a nonstick grill pan over medium heat. Season and pan-fry steak for 20 minutes, or until steak reaches desired doneness. Set aside.

2. Season peppers with salt and pepper. Cook peppers in the same grill pan for about 15 minutes, stirring constantly.

3. Serve steak and peppers immediately.

Turkey and Lettuce Taco Wraps

Serving: 6-8

Total time taken: 30 minutes

Ingredients

- 1 pound lean ground turkey
- ⅔ cups water
- 1 can black beans
- 1 red onion (diced)
- 1 packet taco seasoning
- ½ cup black olives (sliced)
- 1 ½ cup tomatoes (diced)
- 1 ½ cup bell peppers (diced)
- 1 ½ cup corn (diced)
- 1 ½ cup red onion (diced)
- 12 romaine lettuce leaves
- 2 cups Mexican cheese (shredded)
- 1 cup sour cream
- 2 jalapeño peppers (minced)
- 2 cloves of garlic (minced)
- 1 teaspoon rice vinegar
- 1 teaspoon tamari
- 3 scallions (thinly sliced)
- 3 tablespoons cilantro (chopped)
- Hot sauce (for topping)

Directions

1. In a nonstick skillet over medium-high heat, sauté the turkey. Season with salt, pepper, and taco seasoning.

2. When almost cooked, add in jalapeño, garlic, and onion and sauté. Add in the beans and cook until onions are translucent.

3. Stir in rice vinegar and tamari. Cook until the liquid is reduced.

4. To serve, stack two leaves together and top with a spoon of taco filling. Add desired vegetables and sour cream. Garnish with cheese and cilantro.

Zesty Salsa Verde Tacos

Serving: 6

Total time taken: 8 hours 30 minutes

Ingredients

- 2-3 pounds pork roast
- 5 cloves garlic (minced)
- 2 large onion (chopped)
- 3 jars salsa verde
- 2 large avocados (chopped)
- 2 cups lettuce (chopped)
- 2 tomatoes (chopped)
- 1 cup cheese (grated)
- ½ cup green onions (thinly sliced)
- 12-18 corn tortillas
- Salt and pepper, to taste

Directions

1. Set temperature of a 5 quart crock pot to high. Layer onions on the bottom of crock pot.

2. Season pork with salt and pepper, to taste. Layer above onions. Add minced garlic and salsa verde. Cover and cook for 6-8 hours, or until pork pulls apart easily.

3. When pork is cooked, shred the meat. Set aside.

4. To serve, top corn tortillas with pork and choices of vegetables and sour cream.

Wok Veggie Stir Fry

Serving: 4

Total time taken: 55 minutes

Ingredients

- 1 lb boneless chicken breast (cubed)
- 1 teaspoon tomato sauce
- 1 tablespoon olive oil
- 7-8 pieces baby corn
- 1 red bell pepper (sliced)
- 1 green bell pepper (sliced)
- 1 cup cauliflower
- 1 carrot (sliced)
- ½ can mushrooms
- Salt and pepper, to taste

Directions

1. Heat up olive oil over high heat in a large wok. Add the chicken, stirring constantly for 10 minutes until cooked. Remove from wok.

2. Add carrots and cauliflower to the wok. After a few minutes, add the baby corn, mushrooms, peppers, and tomato sauce. Cook for 5-7 minutes.

3. Do not overcook the vegetables, to maintain crispiness.

4. Add the chicken to the wok to heat thoroughly.

5. Serve immediately with rice.

Ricotta and Turkey Sausage Pie

Serving: 8

Total time taken: 35 minutes

Ingredients

- 1 refrigerated pie crust
- 4 eggs
- 2 cups mozzarella cheese (shredded)
- 1 container ricotta cheese
- 1 onion (finely chopped)
- 1 package frozen spinach (chopped)
- Salt and pepper, to taste

Directions

1. Preheat oven to 350 F.

2. Cover a 9-inch pie plate with the rolled-out pie crust. Set aside in refrigerator.

3. Cook sausage in a nonstick skillet, over medium-high heat. Stir constantly until thoroughly cooked, about 8-10 minutes. Drain and clean of excess fat.

4. In a mixing bowl, beat together eggs, salt, and pepper. Add in mozzarella, ricotta, onions, spinach, and sausage. Stir well. Apply mixture into pie crust.

5. Bake for 40-45 minutes, or until an inserted knife comes out clean.

Italian Style Chicken

Serving: 2

Total time taken: 30 minutes

Ingredients

- 4 boneless chicken breasts
- 1 cup chicken broth
- 3 cups sliced mushrooms
- 1 teaspoon italian seasoning
- 1 teaspoon paprika
- Salt and pepper, to taste

Directions

1. Mix italian seasoning, paprika, salt, and pepper together in a bowl. Rub the chicken with the seasoning mix.

2. In a skillet over medium heat, add chicken. Cook until each side is browned, about 3 minutes per side.

3. Add mushrooms and broth into the skillet. Reduce heat, cover, and cook for 20 minutes.

Spicy Chicken Chili

Serving: 2

Total time taken: 3 hours

Ingredients

- 6 cups cooked chicken breasts (diced)
- 2 cups chicken broth
- 1 lb northern beans
- 2 onions (chopped)
- 2 cloves garlic (minced)
- 2 jalapenos (diced)
- 2 chili peppers (diced)
- 1 cup salsa
- 1 teaspoon olive oil
- 2 teaspoons cumin
- ¼ teaspoon cayenne pepper
- 1½ teaspoons oregano

Directions

1. In a large pot, add beans, chicken broth, 1 onion, and 1 minced garlic clove. Simmer for 2 hours, until the beans are soft.

2. In a skillet over medium heat, saute 1 onion, 1 garlic, peppers, cumin, oregano, and cayenne pepper for 5 minutes.

3. Add sauteed peppers, salsa and cooked chicken into the pot. Simmer an additional hour.

4. Serve with cheese or sour cream, as preferred.

Grilled Lemon Shrimp and Spinach Pasta

Serving: 4-6

Total time taken: 30 minutes

Ingredients

- ½ pound large shrimp (shelled and deveined0
- 1 lemon (zested and juiced)
- ⅓ cup half and half (fat free)
- ¼ cup mascarpone cheese
- ¼ cup Parmesan cheese
- ¼ cup toasted pine nuts
- 5 cups baby spinach
- ½ pound whole grain angel hair pasta
- 2 cloves garlic (minced)
- ¼ freshly grated nutmeg
- 1 tablespoon butter (melted)
- Salt and pepper, to taste

Directions

1. Preheat the grill. Marinate the shrimp with lemon zest, lemon juice, butter, salt, pepper, and garlic. Toss and let sit for 30 minutes.

2. Thread shrimp on bamboo skewers, leaving a ¼" space between each shrimp.

3. Grill the skewers for about 6-8 minutes, or until shrimp is opaque. Turn once while grilling.

4. Whisk mascarpone, half and half, and nutmeg in a bowl. Cook over low heat, adding cooked pasta into the sauce.

5. Add spinach and toss. When the spinach wilts, add salt and pepper to taste.

6. For serving, top with Parmesan cheese, grilled shrimp, and pine nuts. Serve immediately.

Walnut Crusted Maple Salmon

Serving: 6

Total time taken: 30 minutes

ngredients

- 2 ½ pounds Alaskan salmon fillets
- 1 teaspoon Worcestershire sauce
- ⅓ cup maple syrum
- ½ teaspoon ground mustard
- ½ cup walnuts
- 2 tablespoons butter
- Cooking spray
- Salt and pepper, to taste
- Lemon wedges (for serving)

Directions

1. Preheat grill to medium heat.

2. In a medium saucepan, melt butter with Worcestershire sauce, maple syrup, mustard, salt, and pepper over medium heat. Warm for about 3-4 minutes. Set aside and let marinade cool to room temperature.

3. In a sealable bag, marinate the salmon for at least 30 minutes.

4. Toast walnuts in a dry skillet, tossing frequently until golden. Roughly chop the walnuts.

5. On a double sheet of foil coated with cooking spray, place marinated salmon. Top with chopped walnuts and salt. Seal foil around the salmon.

6. Grill the aluminum salmon packets for about 10 minutes, or until salmon flakes easily.

7. Serve immediately with lemon wedges.

Grilled Portobello Burger

Serving: 4

Total time taken: 35 minutes

Ingredients

- 4 Portobello mushroom caps
- 4 slices provolone cheese
- 2 tablespoons olive oil
- ¼ cup balsamic vinegar
- 1 tablespoon garlic (minced)
- 1 teaspoon dried basil
- 1 teaspoon dried oregano
- Salt and pepper, to taste

Directions

1. In a shallow baking pan, place mushrooms rounded side up.

2. Whisk oil, vinegar, garlic, basil, oregano, salt, and pepper in a small bowl. Pour over the mushrooms. Let mushrooms sit in marinade for about 15 minutes, turning them halfway through.

3. Preheat grill to medium-high heat. Grill the mushrooms, basting or brushing them with marinade frequently.

4. During last 2 minutes of grilling, top with provolone cheese until melted.

5. Serve immediately on a whole-wheat bun or between lettuce.

Slow-Cooked Beef and Mushrooms

Serving: 2

Total time taken: 8 hours

Ingredients

- 1 lb lean stew beef
- 8 oz mushrooms (sliced)
- ½ cup water
- 1 can cream of mushroom soup
- 1 packet onion soup mix

Directions

1. In a skillet over medium heat, brown the meat.

2. In a slow cooker, add browned meat, mushrooms, soup mix, soup, and water. Cover.

3. Set slow cooker temperature to low. Cook for 8 hours.

4. Serve warm, over noodles or rice.

Parmesan Crusted Tilapia

Serving: 2

Total time taken: 10 minutes

Ingredients

- 2 tilapia fillets
- 2 teaspoons plain yogurt
- 2 teaspoons mayonnaise
- 4 sprigs fresh dill
- ¼ cup parmesan cheese (grated)
- 1 teaspoon garlic powder
- Salt and pepper, to taste
- Cooking spray

Directions

1. Heat oven to broil. Line a baking sheet with aluminum foil and coat with cooking spray.

2. In a bowl, mix yogurt, mayonnaise, and cheese. Mix well.

3. Arrange tilapia on baking sheet. Spread parmesan mixture on each fillet. Sprinkle fillets with dill, garlic powder, and pepper.

4. Cook until fish flakes easily, about 5-7 minutes. (The fish is not necessarily done once the cheese starts browning.)

5. When fish is cooked, turn off broiler. Leave fish in oven for 5 more minutes.

6. Remove from the oven. Serve fish immediately with choice of side.

Turkey Cheddar Veggie Salad

Serving: 6

Total time taken: 30 minutes

ngredients

- 1 lb ground turkey
- 2 tablespoons olive oil
- 1 cup arugula (chopped)
- ½ cup cheddar cheese (grated)
- 1 tomato (finely chopped)
- 1 zucchini (finely chopped)
- ½ cup mushrooms (sliced)
- ¼ teaspoon ground red pepper
- Salt and pepper, to taste.

Directions

1. In a grill pan over medium-high heat, cook ground turkey until brown, about 5 minutes.

2. Add zucchini, mushrooms, salt, and pepper, cooking for 7 minutes. Stir occasionally. Set aside once cooked.

3. In a large bowl, combine arugula, tomato, turkey veggie mix, salt, and pepper. Mix well.

4. Top with cheddar cheese to serve.

Gastric Sleeve Snacks and Dips

Summertime Three-Cheese Vegetable Frittata

Serving: 4

Total time taken: 40 minutes

Ingredients

- ½ cup seeded tomato (chopped)
- ⅓ cup onion (chopped)
- 2 cloves garlic (minced)
- ⅓ cup red bell pepper (chopped)
- ½ cup zucchini (diced)
- 1 tablespoon fresh thyme (chopped)
- 9 large eggs
- ½ tablespoon olive oil
- Salt and pepper, to taste

Directions

1. Preheat broiler.

2. Heat olive oil in broiler-proof skillet. Sauté onion, garlic, bell pepper, zucchini, thyme. Season with salt and pepper. Cover and cook until vegetables are tender, about 7 minutes. Stir occasionally.

3. Stir in the tomato. Cook uncovered until the liquid evaporates, or about 5 minutes.

4. In medium bowl, whisk eggs, salt, and pepper. Pour over the vegetables, stirring gently.

5. Lower the heat and continue to cook. Stir until the eggs are almost set.

6. Cover with aluminum foil and place in broiler until set, about 3 minutes. Serve in wedges.

Avocado in Spicy Sauce

Serving: 2

Total time taken: 30 minutes

Ingredients

- 1 avocado (chopped)
- 1 tablespoon ground curry
- 1 teaspoon soy sauce
- 2 tablespoons olive oil
- ¼ cup water
- ¼ teaspoon red pepper flakes
- 1 teaspoon parsley (finely chopped)
- ¼ teaspoon sea salt

Directions

1. In a large saucepan, heat olive oil over medium-high heat. Add water, ground curry, soy sauce, red pepper, salt, and parsley. Cook for about 5 minutes, stirring occasionally.

2. Add chopped avocado. Stir well and cook until all liquid evaporates, about 3 minutes.

3. Cover saucepan and remove from heat. Let it stand, covered, for 20 minutes before serving.

Mediterranean Red Pepper Dip

Serving: 4

Total time taken: 20 minutes

Ingredients

- 2 oz roasted red pepper
- 2 oz Feta cheese
- ¼ cup hummus
- 1 tablespoon olive oil

Directions

1. In a blender, add roasted red pepper, feta, and hummus.

2. Blend until smooth, adding water or olive oil to reach a desired consistency.

3. Serve with pita chips for a side dip.

Gastric Sleeve Desserts

Mixed Berry Cheesecake Parfait

Serving: 4

Total time taken: 15 minutes

Ingredients

- 6 oz fat-free cream cheese (at room temperature)
- 1 ½ cup plain Greek yogurt
- 3 tablespoons unsalted butter (melted)
- 4 tablespoons sugar
- Seeds from 1 vanilla bean
- Blueberries
- Blackberries
- Strawberries (sliced)
- 1 ¼ cup graham crackers (crushed)
- Mint (for garnish)

Directions

1. Using a food processor, pulse graham crackers until fine. Add melted butter and mix well, until the crumbs are moist. Set aside.

2. Using a stand mixer with a whisk attachment, whip the Greek yogurt, cream cheese, sugar, and vanilla until creamy and smooth.

3. Assemble by layering with graham cracker crumbs, berries, cheesecake filling. Repeat.

4. For garnish, sprinkle on top with berries, graham cracker crumbs, and a mint leaf.

5. Chill for an hour in the refrigerator before serving.

Chocolate and Almond Meringue Cookies

Serving: 24

Total time taken: 2 hours 45 minutes

Ingredients

- ¼ cup unsweetened cocoa
- ½ cup dark chocolate chunks
- ¼ teaspoon vanilla extract
- ¼ teaspoon almond extract
- ½ cup sugar
- ¼ teaspoon salt
- ¼ teaspoon cream of tartar
- 4 egg whites

Directions

1. Preheat oven to 250 F.

2. Using a mixer at high speed, beat egg whites until foamy. Add salt and cream of tartar. Continue to beat until soft peaks form.

3. Add sugar gradually, 1 spoonful at a time, until peaks are stiff. Fold in cocoa, almond extract, and vanilla extract.

4. Cover a baking sheet with parchment paper. Drop spoonfuls of batter onto the baking sheet.

5. Reduce oven temperature to 225 F. Bake until cookies are dry, or about 1½ hours. Turn off oven and let the meringues cool inside the oven for 1 hour.

6. Finish cooling completely on a wire rack.

7. For the glaze, heat chocolate chunks while stirring continuously. When melted, dip half of each meringue into chocolate. Place on wire rack to dry.

8. For storage, keep in an airtight container.

Cinnamon Pumpkin Pudding

Serving: 4

Total time taken: 15 minutes

Ingredients

- 4 cups unsweetened pumpkin juice
- 1 lb pumpkin (chopped)
- 1 cup orange juice
- 2 tablespoons honey
- ½ cup cornstarch
- 3 ground cloves
- 1 teaspoon cinnamon

Directions

1. In a bowl, combine pumpkin juice, orange juice, honey, cornstarch, cloves, and cinnamon.

2. In a large pot, add the pumpkin pieces and pumpkin juice mixture. Stir well. Heat over medium heat until almost boiling.

3. Reduce heat to low and cook until thickened, about 15 minutes.

4. Pour into bowls immediately. Set aside to completely cool. Chill for at least 15 minutes in refrigerator before serving.

Bariatric Smoothies and Juices

Banana & Strawberry Protein Smoothie

Serving: 1

Total time taken: 10

Ingredients

- 1 ¼ strawberries (sliced)
- 1 banana
- 10 almonds
- 3 tablespoons protein powder (chocoolate)
- Ice cubes

Directions

1. In a blender, mix strawberries, banana, almonds, and water.

2. Add ice cubes, blend.

3. Add protein powder, blend.

4. Continue to mix until well-blended, about 30 seconds.

Minty Pineapple Raspberry Juice

Serving: 1

Total time taken: 10 minnutes

Ingredients

- 1 cup rasberries (chopped)
- 1 cup pineapples (chopped)
- 1 tablespoon honey
- 1 cup lemon juice
- 1 cup mint leaves
- ½ teaspoon salt

Directions

1. Use blender to extract juice from pineapples and raspberries.

2. Add juices and lemon juice to a pitcher.

3. Add in salt and honey until well combined.

4. Crush mint leaves, adding them to juice.

5. Serve cold.

Coconut Ginger Peach Smoothie

Serving: 4

Total time taken: 10 minutes

Ingredients

- 1 peach (chopped)
- 1 cup coconut milk
- 1 tablespoon chia seeds
- 1 tablespoon fresh ginger (chopped)
- 1 tablespoon coconut oil
- Ice cubes

Directions

1. Clean, cut, and prepare all ingredients.

2. In a blender, combine coconut milk, peach, ginger, and coconut oil. Blend until smooth.

3. Pour smoothie into a serving glass. Stir in chia seeds.

4. Serve with ice and garnish with mint leaves.

Avocado Cherry Breakfast Smoothie

Serving: 3

Total time taken: 10 minutes

Ingredients

- 1 cup coconut water
- 1 lime
- 1 cup fresh cherries
- ½ avocado (chopped)
- Ice cubes

Directions

1. Clean, cut, and prepare all ingredients.

2. In a blender, combine coconut water, cherries, avocado, and lime. Blend until smooth.

3. Pour into a serving glass with ice. Refrigerate for 10 minutes and then serve.

Vanilla Mango Smoothie

Serving: 3

Total time taken: 10 minutes

Ingredients

- 1 cup coconut milk
- 1 mango (chopped)
- 1 teaspoon vanilla extract
- 1 tablespoon walnuts (chopped)
- Ice cubes

Directions

1. Clean, cut, and prepare all ingredients.

2. In a blender, combine coconut milk, mango, vanilla extract, and walnuts. Blend until smooth.

3. Pour into glasses with ice cubes. Serve immediately.

Healthy Green Smoothie

Serving: 2

Total time taken: 10 minutes

Ingredients

- 1 cup water
- ½ cup kale (chopped)
- 1 cup white grapes
- 3 tablespoons green tea powder
- 1 tablespoon honey
- ½ teaspoon fresh mint (ground)

Directions

1. Clean, cut, and prepare all ingredients.

2. Dissolve green tea powder into 2 tablespoons of hot water for 2 minutes. Set aside.

3. In a blender, combine water, kale, grapes, honey, and mint. Blend until smooth. Stir in tea mixture.

4. Pour into glasses. Refrigerate for 30 minutes and then serve.

Banana Guava Smoothie

Serving: 2

Total time taken: 10 minutes

Ingredients

- 2 cups water
- 1 cup guava (chopped)
- 1 banana (sliced)
- 1 cup baby spinach (chopped)
- ½ mango (chopped)
- 1 teaspoon fresh ginger (grated)

Directions

1. Clean, cut, and prepare all ingredients.

2. In a blender, combine banana, guava, mango, spinach, and ginger. Gradually add water and blend until creamy.

3. Pour into serving glasses. Refrigerate for 20 minutes and then serve.

Grape Raspberry Refresher

Serving:1

Total time taken: 10 minutes

Ingredients

- 1 cup raspberries (chopped)
- 1 cup grapes (chopped)
- 1 teaspooon honey
- 1 cup lemon juice
- Mint leaves
- Ice cubes
- ½ teaspoon salt

Directions

1. Use blender to extract juice from grapes and raspberries.

2. Mix with lemon juice, salt, and honey until well combined.

3. Serve cold atop ice cubes. Garnish with mint leaves.

Detox Smoothie

Serving: 2

Total time taken: 10 minutes

Ingredients

- 1 banana (chopped)
- 1 cup baby spinach (chopped)
- ½ avocado (chopped)
- 1 tablespoon goji berries
- 1 tablespoon flaxseed (ground)
- 1 teaspoon turmeric (ground)
- 1 tablespoon stevia
- Ice cubes

Directions

1. Clean, cut, and prepare all ingredients.

2. In a blender, combine banana, spinach, avocado, turmeric, flaxseed. Blend until smooth.

3. Pour into serving glasses with ice. Serve cold.

Creamy Cucumber Protein Smoothie

Serving: 2

Total time taken: 10 minutes

Ingredients

- ¼ cup Greek yogurt
- 1 serving vanilla protein powder
- ¼ cup skim milk
- 1 ounce cucumber (cubed)
- 1½ tablespoon applesauce
- ⅛ teaspoon cinnamon
- Liquid stevia, to taste
- Ice cubes

Directions

1. In a blender, combine yogurt, milk, cucumber, applesauce, and cinnamon. Add liquid stevia to taste.

2. Blend until smooth.

3. Pour into serving glasses with ice. Serve cold.

Cinnamon Toast Smoothie

Serving: 2

Total time taken: 10 minutes

Ingredients

- ¼ cup cottage cheese
- ¼ cup skim milk
- 2 oz frozen skim milk cubes
- 1 serving vanilla protein powder
- ⅛ teaspoon butter extract
- ¼ teaspoon cinnamon
- Dash of nutmeg
- Liquid stevia, to taste

Directions

1. Fill an ice cube tray with skim milk. Freeze overnight.

2. In a blender, add milk cubes, cottage cheese, milk, protein powder, butter extract, cinnamon, and nutmeg. Add liquid stevia to taste.

3. Blend until smooth. Serve cold.

Four Stage Meal Plan

There are four stages for a Gastric Sleeve Post-Op Diet, as explained in our earlier chapter. There are recipes in this book suited for all four stages and beyond. In this chapter, we will break down which recipes will help you during the stages, so that you can decide what meal is best suited for your diet.

This is a quick reminder of the four stages.

Phase 1: Clear Liquids: first 1-2 weeks

Phase 2: Full Liquid: next 1-2 weeks

Phase 3: Soft Pureed Food: next 1-4 weeks

Phase 4 Soft Foods and Beyond

Phase 1: Clear Liquids:

In the first 1-2 weeks after you have cleared the hospital, the goal is to sip 1 ounce of fluids in 15 minutes. This is meant to control your initial intake of food and drinks. This period is crucial to getting your body to understand the new routine. You can only consume clear liquids at this point, which all are easily available in any grocery store. During this stage, you are only allowed the following:

- Water
- Ice cubes
- Broth
    - Low Sodium Chicken Broth
    - Low Sodium Beef Broth
    - Vegetable Broth
- Sugar Free popsicles or jello

- Sugar free juice or beverage
  - Coconut water
  - Diluted fruit juice
  - Sugar free Kool Aid

Phase 2: Full Liquids:

The following 1-2 weeks you can go into a full liquid diet. The goal is to get about 70-85 grams per day, 50-70 ounces of fluid per day, and between 500-600 calories per day. It is important to get a lot of liquids in your system during this time to prevent dehydration and constipation. During this stage, all liquids consumed need to be thinner than a milk shake so that it's is easy for your stomach to consume. The following are what is allowed to be eaten:

- Everything from Phase 1
- Protein drinks
- Fat-free milk or soy milk
- Light yogurt
- Reduced Fat soups (see our soup & liquid recipes chapters)
  - Blended pea soup
  - Minestrone soup
  - Bell Pepper Basil Soup (no tomato)
  - Soup with White beans
  - Cream of Chicken & Rice Soup
- Smoothie and light juices (see our smoothie & juice chapter)

Phase 3: Soft Pureed Food:

Once you are at the 2 week mark after your surgery, your doctor will most likely recommend you to approach phase 3 of your diet journey. Soft Pureed Food means mostly blended and easily chewable foods. The goal is still about 70-85 grams per day, with 50-70 ounces of fluid per day. One should aim for 3-4 servings of food per day, with liquid in between meals. Liquids should not be consumed within 30 meals of a meal. The following foods and recipes are suitable for the phase 3 diet.

- Everything from Phase 1 & 2
- Low fat cheese
- Pureed meats
- Tofu
- Mash potatoe
- Baby food
- Mashed Veggies
- Everything form the Smoothie and juice chapter
- Everything from the Sauce chapter
- Everything from the Soup chapter
- Everything in the Puree chapter

Phase 4 Soft Foods and Beyond

At this point, you are ready for soft foods and very soon regular food. This stage will ease you back to the normal foods you eat, but with several exceptions. You can select pretty much every recipe in this book. However, remember the following important rules:

- Start with Veggie & Soup recipes before moving on to heavier items
- Always avoid sugar, especially in sauces and liquids
- Choose low fat or low protein foods
- Always eat slowly and chew foods well

Always remember to consult your surgeon or doctor as everyone is different and may need a modified diet plan. Ensure that you follow their instructions and follow the diet that is most recommended for you.

Conclusion

Now that you have seen how much potential there is to continue eating delicious, exciting meals after bariatric surgery, you are in a better place to enjoy your new life on the diet. As the weight continues to shift, aim to pull as many different recipes into your diet as possible. This will ensure that you are getting a maximum amount of nutrients and vitamins.

Keep the information on goals and limits front of mind whenever you are cooking ordering, and eating. If you're ever in doubt, contact your doctor or seek support from the many bariatric communities out there.

Take the information in this book one recipe at a time. Adjusting to life post-surgery isn't a race, nor should the many recipes be a source of panic. As you become more comfortable with what works for you, you will be able to tailor the recipes to make the diet work for you, and not the other way around.

Printed in Great Britain
by Amazon

87170145R00086